T0124106

EBURY PRESS

MOVEMINT MEDICINE

Dr Rajat Chauhan is a student of running (for the past thirty-seven years) and pain. He is the founder and race director of La Ultra, an epic ultramarathon held in Ladakh since 2010. It features categories from 11 km to 555 km across altitudes varying from 11,000 feet to 17,700 feet. Dr Chauhan is the author of *La Ultra: cOuch to 5, 11 & 22 km in 100 days*, and has been a columnist for *Mint* and *Hindustan Times*. He got his MBBS degree from Manipal College of Medical Sciences, Pokhara, Nepal, and his MSc degree in sports-exercise medicine from Queen's Medical Centre, Nottingham, UK. This was followed by a membership of the London College of Osteopathic Medicine. He was founding head, sports medicine department, Manipal Hospital, Bangalore, and founding director, sports department, Ashoka University. He was the (quit) chairperson of the World Congress of Science and Medicine in Cricket, held during the 2011 Cricket World Cup which was hosted by India, and the principal running technical consultant and head coach for Adidas India. He is a senior fellow at Livonics Institute of Integrated Learning and Research.

Dr Darren J. Player is a scientist and an academic. He studied personal training, exercise referral and sports science before completing his PhD in muscle cellular and molecular physiology. Dr Player has also undertaken professional qualifications in nutritional coaching and sports massage. He is an external examiner for a UK Sport Science degree and personal training qualifications. Combining his scientific background and professional qualifications, he has a unique view of health, fitness and exercise. A published author, he has contributed chapters in two scientific textbooks and has published numerous articles in prestigious scientific journals. Dr Player has also been invited to speak at scientific conferences and acclaimed academic and medical institutions, including AIIMS, IIT Delhi and the University of Washington. As a teenager, he was a competitive 200-metre and 400-metre runner. Now he just trains for health and well-being.

ALSO BY DR RAJAT CHAUHAN

The Pain Handbook

'As doctors, we are often made to think that we are gods. We are taught how to treat disease, how to do surgeries and how to fix broken bones. We are not taught how to create health. I started my health journey eight years back, late by any standards, at the age of forty-eight years. And I feel the fittest now, more than ever in my life. I am grateful to know Dr Rajat Chauhan, who convinced me that I didn't have a major problem when I was advised a knee replacement, who lifted my morale when it was at rock bottom after years of pain and who told me that I would be able to run a marathon one day. Yoga happened by chance. I was desperately looking for solutions as medicine did not give me any. Yoga taught me that health is very simple and doable; it's the disease that should be difficult. I wish Rajat and Darren all the best for this beautiful book and I feel blessed to be part of it'—Dr Anjali Kumar, senior consultant gynaecologist and obstetrician and founder, Maitri, a digital platform on women's health

'Life has become too hectic to think about all the steps to good health and fitness. This book gives you a blueprint written in a very innovative and interesting way. It's a must-read for professionals and laymen alike who are looking to improve their health and fitness holistically'—Vesna Peričević Jacob, holistic fitness guru and founder, Vesna's Alta Celo

'I shied away from accepting what I suspected—my mental state was dictated by my physical state. This book helped me unshackle myself. I am what I do, eat and sleep!'—Manish Sharma, co-founder, Printo, mountaineer and ultrarunner

MOVEMINT
MEDICINE

YOUR JOURNEY TO PEAK HEALTH

DR RAJAT CHAUHAN
DR DARREN PLAYER

EBURY
PRESS

An imprint of Penguin Random House

EBURY PRESS

USA | Canada | UK | Ireland | Australia
New Zealand | India | South Africa | China

Ebury Press is part of the Penguin Random House group of companies
whose addresses can be found at global.penguinrandomhouse.com

Published by Penguin Random House India Pvt. Ltd
4th Floor, Capital Tower 1, MG Road,
Gurugram 122 002, Haryana, India

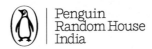

First published in Ebury Press by Penguin Random House India 2022

Text and Illustrations copyright © Rajat Chauhan and Darren Player 2022
Illustrations by Archana Rajgopal

ISBN 9780143453000

Typeset in Adobe Caslon Pro by Manipal Technologies Limited, Manipal

www.penguin.co.in

Dedicated to Mummy and Papa; Nidhi, Harsheath and Viren; 'La Ultra' and 'Run & Bee' family; and formal and informal mentors, all who have consulted me for pain, sports or running, each in their different ways have shown me that there is no one way to get off your arse and move that tiny bit more. And to Darren for being my partner in crime during my darkest phase in life.

—Dr Rajat Chauhan

To Meena, who has sat for hours listening to my ramblings and thoughts about the book, and loves and supports me in everything I do. To my two children, who keep me grounded and make me appreciate everything in life. To my parents, who gave me so many opportunities when I was growing up and who still support me today.
Finally, to Rajat, as a colleague and mentor, but also a close friend and supporter.

—Dr Darren Player

Contents

Introduction

Students for Life

In March 2019, Darren James Player was in Delhi for a research visit. Dr Kshitij Malik, a member of the University College London (UCL) Alumni Network, invited him for dinner and asked if he could bring a friend along. This friend was Rajat Chauhan, a senior from Manipal College of Medical Sciences, Pokhara, Nepal.

It became evident very early on at the dinner (in fact, it was probably before drinks had been served) that we—Darren and Rajat—shared many values. Not only did we know many of the same people (sport and exercise medicine is a small world!), but we also felt very strongly that an alternative approach was required to both treat patients and advise the general public about exercise.

The following conversation was similar to the one we had when we first met, and it sums up why this book is in your hands today.

* * *

Where did it all start for you, Rajat?

Rajat: I'm from a small village in Delhi that dates back to 1202 CE. History followed me to Wynberg-Allen School tucked away in Mussoorie, a quaint hill station in the Himalayas. The sports teacher would run behind us at 5 a.m. and cane the boy who came last. At that point, the aim was to come second to last to avoid the caning, but the goalposts soon moved.

Every fortnight, the top six runners won a mango drink. Therefore, my goal quickly changed from wanting to come second to last to coming sixth. As time went by, I started running a little faster on weekends to get that drink because pocket money used to be Rs 25 and the drink used to be worth Rs 2. So, you could effectively earn extra pocket money by doing well in the races.

When I moved to Delhi, I wanted to pick up running as a career, but my parents were not particularly keen on the idea. They were pleased that I had a passion for running and that it was a great practice from the point of view of health, but they were clear that it did not pay the bills! I appreciated their perspective, even if I did not like it at the time, and so, I went along with what they wanted for me and studied medicine.

How about you, Darren? How did you end up where you are? Was it a story that was carved out for you from an early age?

Darren: I was always active as a child and very fortunate that my parents encouraged and supported my involvement in many sports and societies. In fact, I soon realized—as early as primary school—that I was a fast runner. I would excel during sports day and other such events. When I got to senior school, I was still one of the fastest among my peers (and even among seniors) and was encouraged to take part in athletics. At inter-school events, both local and regional, I would compete in 200-m and 400-m races, finishing among the top three in most cases. This would often make my schoolmates ask whether I was destined for the Olympics, a thought that stayed with me for a long time.

Although it was a 'niggling' thing in the back of my mind, when competing at the regional club level, I realized that I would need to be a lot better than I was if I were to make it to the Olympics. That's when I thought about a different path in life.

Academic studies were always a little harder for me. I never felt particularly motivated or interested in most subjects. I did reasonably well in secondary school and finished with As (almost all) at the GCSE level (standard qualification in secondary school). After this, it was predicted that I would score straight As at A-Level (higher qualification in secondary school), which, deep down, was something that I did not think I could ever achieve.

At this point I was torn. Was I to pursue a career in the police force or continue with academic studies in an area that was of interest to me? A friend's mother shared a newspaper article with me about opportunities within the police if one entered the force after completing a degree. This could be any degree. So, it meant that I could study a subject that I was passionate about—sport and exercise.

There was a lot of pressure (mainly from teachers) to apply to well-known and established courses at universities with long-standing reputations. However, I wanted to study a practical course that was relevant to clinical populations. With this in mind, I opted for a brand-new course at a relatively small university—University of Bedfordshire, formerly De Montfort University, UK. I chose to study for a degree in Exercise and Fitness Practice (Sport and Exercise Science with additional vocational qualifications). In the end, I did not get the grades that I was expected to achieve at A-Level. In a way, it was good that I decided not to opt for some of the universities that were asking for higher grades! Every journey happens for a reason.

This degree course that I decided to pursue was the first of its kind in the UK. The idea was to combine the academic disciplines of sport and exercise with practical qualifications in fitness instructing, personal training and exercise referral. Many other universities now use this approach as it provides 'added value' to an academic degree and allows students to work with clients and patients to apply theoretical knowledge. It is a shame that after more than 15 years of such courses being in existence, they are still not recognized and appreciated to the level that they should be.

What was your experience when you were in medical school, Rajat?

Rajat: By my second year, I wanted to quit. Dr Hardev Singh Girn, a friend's dad, told me that my situation was similar to being in the middle of a river. If I swam back, I would have no degree, but if I crossed it, I would at least have one. Sadly, he was right. With a degree, I would have the choice to either practise medicine or do whatever else I wanted with my life. So, I decided to just carry on with finishing medical college.

I found that in the beginning, my batchmates—all good people—were very excited about treating patients with empathy. As we started working with clinical subjects—the time when you really start seeing patients—I saw that they had somehow become indifferent to people in general. It was all about grades. I suspect the system is to be blamed where the focus is to pass exams because there is just so much to cover. My batchmates had markedly reduced empathy for patients or were, by then, simply lacking it. I found them to be a lot ruder, a characteristic that had somehow gotten attached to their professional personalities. The only mission ahead of them was to pass exams, and for some, it was to top them. I am probably being too judgemental, but in his book, *Gesundheit!: Bringing Good Health to You, the Medical System, and Society through Physician Service, Complementary Therapies, Humor, and Joy*, Dr Patch Adams talks about six characteristics of a good doctor: happy, funny, loving, cooperative, creative and thoughtful.[1] I found them missing in my friends. Several studies have now reported this phenomenon all across the world. Empathy, a basic human characteristic, gradually starts dwindling as students advance in their medical studies. The system is such that the best of us end up becoming another brick in the wall.

Even when it came to knowing more about the people (patients), their backgrounds and medical problems, my friends from medical college would memorize questions from the books, while the conversation with the patient (person) would be very mechanical. Care was missing. Patients weren't allowed to tell their stories. They simply weren't given that time. There was no eagerness to understand the human being.

In medical college, the first patient we end up seeing is a dead body (a cadaver). It teaches us a lot, but it can't narrate its story, move, feel or think, whereas the ones we cater to eventually as doctors, do all of this and more. This plays a major role in how we, medical students then and doctors later, treat living people as dead, possibly subconsciously. All we see are medical conditions, not people.

Over the years, I have learnt that if we let people talk, they will offer solutions to their own problems. It could very well come after an hour of conversation or after a few consultations. I totally love the Sherlock Holmes-like role that consultations involve. I so envy the 4–5-hour first consultations that Dr Adams used to do.

In any case, the focus throughout medical school was on illness and sickness, whereas what came instinctively to me was health and wellness. As an athlete, you are interested in performing at the optimal level. I was far ahead in that space compared to my batchmates because I had a head start of almost a decade over them since I had been running from the age of nine. I knew what it took to float without trying to breathe. I was combining art and science long before anyone would talk to me about it. My peers had no clue what they were missing out on. Pathology (the science of the causes and effects of diseases, and especially the branch of medicine that deals with the laboratory examination of samples of body tissue for diagnostic or forensic purposes) was everywhere and there was not enough talk of physiology (the branch of biology that deals with the normal functions of living organisms and their parts). How could these people ever appreciate exercise and movement, leave alone happiness and laughter?

There was more psychology in forensic medicine than in psychiatry. Of course, it was below our dignity to speak about psychology. We were taught about the pharmaceutical approach as that's what would get us to pass exams. No one was talking about Dr Adams' six characteristics. In middle school, I once got a caning on my backside (best of six) because I smiled in class. Beat that, punished for smiling! Not even laughing. For over two decades now, my closing line in all communications is 'Keep miling and smiling'.

What was it like after medical school, Rajat?

Rajat: I wanted to specialize in paediatrics because I'd always loved being around children and their straightforward nature was refreshing. I soon realized that besides being mediocre at medicine, I didn't like how patients were treated like guinea pigs.

The only thing that made sense was doing a master's in sports and exercise medicine, combining my passion and profession. I am glad I made that choice because my course director, Dr Peter L. Gregory, is a gem of a person who soon became a friend and a mentor and has been one ever since. While doing MBBS, we really weren't taught how to do any research or critical thinking. This course had top-notch faculty that delved deep into psychology, nutrition, sleep, exercise and sports. Yet, the dots were left unconnected.

Even though I now had a master's in sports-exercise medicine, I didn't know how to treat patients with my hands. There was a situation where, during a football match where

I was the duty doctor, I simply didn't know what to do. Dr Gregory suggested a course that he said he would have taken up if he had known about it a decade ago.

I was fortunate to be accepted into the London College of Osteopathic Medicine. Most would wonder why someone would pick a course in alternative medicine after having a degree in modern medicine and then a master's too! We were taught to question everything that was taught to us, unlike in my bachelor's. I remember that Dr Roderic Macdonald, the principal at that time, told us that if all we were to learn at the end of the course was that it had all been a total waste of time, it would be worth it. At least we would have learnt what *not* to do. The wonderful tutors taught us to touch and listen, not with our hands and ears but with our hearts.

From medical school to clinics to hospitals, all of them have skeletons hung up somewhere, almost sending a message that that's all we are—a bag full of bones. And that's what most doctors are busy treating—bones and organs—without appreciating what gets them moving. Most of our doctor colleagues have their eyes wide shut and miss seeing that the skull is grinning from ear to ear as it knows a lot more about movement.

What are your thoughts on this, Darren?

Darren: This is a very interesting point, that we often forget or overlook some of the very basic things in science and medicine, even when they are staring right back at us! After graduating, although I had qualified as a personal trainer and was also qualified to work with patients to treat them with exercise, I recognized that there was a huge gap in the 'fitness industry'. I wanted to learn more about how and why exercise was so powerful as a medicine in order to be able to treat patients better, so I continued my academic studies through a PhD.

When I finished my PhD, I continued on the academic path and began my postdoctoral training. When people came to know I had finished my PhD, many of them would joke and say, 'Well, you're not a real doctor, are you?' This was personal, since my brother finished medical school a year before I finished my PhD. I knew that we were both on different career paths, but it certainly got me thinking. What is it that I am doing that can have a positive impact on patients?

I was fortunate enough to work for part of my time as a translational scientist at the National Centre for Sport and Exercise Medicine (Loughborough University, UK). This is a legacy of the UK government from the London 2012 Olympics, aimed at using sport and physical activity to promote health. The opportunity allowed me to go back to what I first enjoyed during my initial studies—developing practical solutions for health impact and working with the public to promote health and well-being. It finally allowed me to use practical knowledge and skills that I had developed some years ago. It also opened my eyes to the challenges of promoting public health messages, especially in communities where certain things are not commonplace.

Engaging with the large South Asian community in Leicestershire (where I was working) was an experience that taught me a lot about public well-being. I remember, on one particular occasion, having to explain the benefits of resistance exercise to a lady who was looking to lose weight. Her mobility was poor, so engaging in resistance exercise would have improved mobility to support walking and other cardio exercises. She did not quite see the merit in this approach, suggesting that she was already strong enough and did not want big biceps! Despite all the scientific knowledge I had, I still had lots to learn (and I still do, to this day) about how to communicate with people and motivate them to develop positive health behaviour.

How about you, Rajat?

Rajat: Same here. My biggest realization is that I'll be a student for life, a student of pain and running.

During weekends, I would attend a lot of certificate and diploma courses that had anything to teach about movement and pain. The tutors were all kinds of professionals ranging from dancers, nurses, physiotherapists, physicians, surgeons and singers. Without an iota of self-importance, I was happy to learn about acupuncture, dry needling, acupressure, taping, spinal injections, Alexander technique, yoga, Pilates, etc. In the mornings, I would often video record my running club members to understand their movements.

While I was at London College of Osteopathic Medicine, Dr Robert Atkins' (famous for the Atkins diet) work in nutrition was rubbished. I happily obliged and jumped on the bandwagon. Looking back at it, I was becoming like Brad Pitt's character in the film *War Machine*: 'Glen was known as a humble man. But humble in a way that says my humility makes me better than you.'[2]

My first job in London, while I was still at London College of Osteopathic Medicine, was at Kieser Training (London), a Swiss-German chain of rehabilitation centres that focused on strength training. I was the head of medical strength training there, catering to neck, back and knee pain. The slogan Kieser Training had back then was 'strong back knows no pain', a very German statement. All my well-intentioned colleagues and tutors from the osteopathic college frowned upon me for suggesting high-intensity, machine-based exercises as treatment for pain. What was being missed out was the fact that Kieser Training worked because we made patients take a proactive, central role in their journey to recovery, unlike the healthcare industry's approach. The patients also built confidence along with some muscles. There was so much psychology at play, a fact that we didn't realize much at the time.

I would often get patients travelling from places that were 3–4 hours away. They would not be able to come as regularly as I would like them to. But their results were on a par with those who were living in London and coming to Kieser Training two to three times a week. It puzzled me for a while. Patients who were disciplined with exercises, be they simple or complicated or whether doing them on machines or on the floor, showed results. Those who weren't disciplined, no matter where they lived and how they did the exercises, were not showing enough results. The big lesson being that a good exercise is one that's done regularly.

I was only able to pick these roles of psychology in exercise courtesy Dr Jens Foell, a German general practitioner practising in London with a special interest in pain. He used to train at Kieser Training. He suggested that I attend weekend modules of a new and upcoming psychology school of thought called Human Givens that was openly questioning the traditional approach to psychology and making it accessible to anyone and everyone. For some odd reason, in all the medical and allied fields, so-called experts want to make everything as complicated as possible to sound more brilliant than they really are.

What are your thoughts on this, Darren?

Darren: Same here! I experienced how certain scientific and medical principles are challenged at a conference in Glasgow during my PhD. Prof. Timothy Noakes was challenging the dogma around what limits exercise performance—is it the muscles, or the heart and lungs? Noakes proposes that there is a 'central governor' within the brain that limits our exercise capacity to protect us and, needless to say, there have been some strong challenges to this hypothesis. I was on the side of most people who would not necessarily agree with Noakes. However, there has been increasing evidence over the years that at least some of what he says may well be true. This has taught me a vital lesson, which is to think broadly and never dismiss something without listening to the full story.

Someone once introduced an analogy to me, which I have tried to emulate. Much like when we try on a new jumper, we first look at it to check if we like the style, colour, shape, etc. We then try on the jumper for size, to check if it fits and feels comfortable. If it does, we buy it; if it doesn't, we put it back on the shelf (or return it to our favourite online store!). We should all take the same approach when it comes to information about health and well-being—look at it, size it up and if you like it, keep it. If not, dismiss it and move on.

Do you share the same sentiment, Rajat?

Rajat: It was at the 2004 Lawn Tennis Association conference (London, UK) that I witnessed, for the first time, how we all could come together to add value to what we knew since we were all busy working in our silos. All kinds of professionals involved in lawn tennis—coaches, trainers, managers, doctors, physiotherapists, players, nutritionists, scientists, etc.,—sat in one room, trying their best to not let their egos come in the way. Easier said than done. Even the best of us suffers from the Glen syndrome (referring to the character from *War Machine*).

At this conference, I was also fortunate to hear Prof. Timothy Noakes who went into the mecca of medicine and then respectfully ripped apart Dr Archibald V. Hill's work for which Hill had received the 1922 Nobel Prize in Physiology or Medicine. Everything Noakes uttered was backed by evidence. Hill had suggested that oxygen is the limiting factor to how long muscles can carry on working in intense conditions, indirectly pointing to the heart. Noakes, on the other hand, proposed for the first time in 1997 that it was the brain that was the 'central governor', helping us work harder but stopping just before we get into a dangerous zone, else we would all die each time we push ourselves hard while doing exercises. There was an uproar in the room. If all those sports exercise medicine and science experts could, they would have murdered Noakes, each of them gleefully waiting for their turn to stab him. But he stood his ground.

I found it really fascinating that the best of experts took this long to make the body-mind connect when Dr Adams had already been at it for over three decades. I fail to understand why they take statements made by Hippocrates more than two millennia ago for granted.

More than five centuries ago, Leonardo da Vinci had said something that some of us have quoted but most of us have forgotten to practise, becoming blind to the obvious: 'Study the science of art. Study the art of science. Develop your senses—especially learn how to see. Realize that everything connects to everything else.'[3] Thanks to Dr Adams, I try to understand the patient, I let them talk. I have become more of a counsellor to them than someone who judges them because they are more than that. They are people with a story that needs to be told and heard.

I connect move (physical activity, exercise, sports, breathing), sleep (rest, recovery), mind (psychology, happiness, smiling, contentment—that there is always a choice to be happy and mentally healthy) and common sense about food, and how all this is further connected to what they are faced with. I make them feel human again. And for that, I am forever grateful to Dr Adams. It is these four essential components for health that we discuss in this book in a unique way, in the hope that you will be inspired to act.

* * *

A Note on the Title

When a dream takes hold of you, what can you do? You can run with it. Let it run your life. Or let it go. And think for the rest of your life, about what might have been.

—Dr Patch Adams[4]

To raise awareness of the benefits of movement, physical activity and exercise, we coined the phrase: *MoveMint Medicine*, a deliberate play on words.

The *verb* 'to move' has a couple of definitions according to the Oxford English Dictionary,[5] some of which we have commented on here:

• To go from one place, position, state, etc., to another.

This obviously relates to the physical nature of *MoveMint*, where we all need to be moving more.

• (intransitive) Of a person or thing: to go, advance, proceed, pass from one place to another.

This relates to the psychological, emotional and general life aspects of *MoveMint Medicine*, where, through exercise, it is possible to see progress, not only in physical terms but in many aspects of life too. Throughout this book, there are many examples of this which will hopefully serve as motivation to you.

There are also a number of meanings to the term 'mint'.[6] As an adjective, 'mint' can be used to describe:

• 'That is in mint condition'; new or as if new.

This reflects the idea that through exercise, it is possible to feel restored and regenerated. There is also some evidence of this anatomically and physiologically, where certain structures and systems can be restored to younger conditions or to how they were before injury or disease.

- (colloquial) Excellent, great.

This is the colloquial or slang use of the adjective 'mint', often used in the UK to describe something as good. This follows that exercise should be fun, exciting and something that we want to do.

As a *noun*, the word 'mint' can also have multiple meanings:

- Any of various aromatic plants constituting the genus Mentha (family: Lamiaceae or Labiatae), which includes many kinds grown as culinary herbs; esp. a cultivated plant of this genus, spec. spearmint, M. spicata.
- Used the world over in food and drinks as well as a medicinal herb, mint is natural and known for its 'fresh' taste. After all, mint is used in toothpastes, chewing gums and other mouth freshening products. *MoveMint* brings a natural and fresh approach to give you a 'breath of fresh air' for your health and well-being.
- An establishment where money is coined, usually under the authority and direction of the state.

The process of making new coins is similar to what we want to advocate with this book. 'Stamping' a mark on your health and well-being in a new way that will last a lifetime.

- (chiefly with of) A quantity of money coined; a vast sum of money. Frequently to make (also lose, etc.) a mint (of money). Also (in extended use): a vast quantity or amount.

The tools that are provided to you in this book will allow you to build your 'bank' of health. This will be an opportunity for you to 'invest' in your health. As they say, 'health is wealth', so it should be the biggest investment you make.

It is also important to consider what 'medicine' actually means and how it is practised in modern society. The goal of the *MoveMint Medicine* initiative is to support and promote an ethical practice of medicine, which puts the patient at the centre. Unfortunately, many doctors and practitioners do not listen to the needs and desires of the patient enough, although the tide is turning in this respect.

The dictionary definitions of 'medicine' provide some good points of discussion for this book.

The *noun* 'medicine' is used in two main contexts:[7]

- The science or practice of the diagnosis, treatment, and prevention of disease (in technical use often taken to exclude surgery).

Although this definition has significance in modern medicine and forms the basis of all medical training, somehow the art of medicine is lost in translation. The art of listening to our patients, having the skills to touch them and having the ability to feel what they are feeling are majorly neglected in the instant gratification practice of medicine. Both patients and doctors are to be blamed for it, along with, of course, the system.

- A substance or preparation used in the treatment of illness; a drug; esp. one taken by mouth.

This definition of medicine is particularly interesting, as it emphasizes the apparent necessity for the use of a drug or 'other preparation'. The term 'other preparation' is ambiguous and could be referring to natural remedies, as would have been the case prior to the advent of the pharmaceutical industry.

* * *

There are four main areas of importance in this book: movement, sleep, nutrition and the mind. These are all dependent on each other for overall health and well-being. On their own, they are nothing. All four are equally important for our overall well-being. It's unfair to say that one is more important than the other. Unfortunately, you'll not find many doctors who touch upon these four, leave alone make a connection between them.

Through all of these, we will make a fresh connection between body, mind and sole. Yes, you read it right. We left out 'soul' because, as humans, we like to buy into any theory that suggests we'll live forever in one way or another.

Our soles help us in the 'now', unlike the 'soul' which promises an obscure idea of a never-ending 'future'. Quite literally, our soles keep us grounded at all times. They make us who we are. We need to be reminded about them repeatedly because we forget and take them for granted.

MoveMint Medicine is about making you aware of how important these are and why you need to be better informed. Passivity, be gone!

As Darren said earlier, try this jumper to see whether it fits. If it does, we would love to hear from you. If it doesn't, we would still love to hear from you.

1

Dream, Life and Patch

A dream.

We've been smitten by a dream, a dream to make all citizens of the whole world become more responsible towards themselves.

Once we all realize that we are CEOs of our complete selves, both the body and the mind, it's game on. This world will be a much better place.

We need to take on the onus of our own health, rather than keep outsourcing it. It is not only our right but a duty to ourselves and our loved ones to become the best versions of ourselves, in every sense. And, it starts with our overall health.

It is no top secret today that the 'healthcare industry' all around the world is failing us, in some places more than others. The flaw is in the system, not in any one person or speciality. We can't just put the blame, rightly or wrongly, on someone else and get on with it. It is, after all, our own life that we can be sure about. So might as well be in control, or as much as we possibly can be.

The term 'healthcare' itself is also a misnomer as even in the best-case scenario the system is addressing illness and sickness, with not much interest in your overall health till you fall sick or ill. Even in sickness, somehow, quality of life is not given as much importance as extending life. It seems the system exploits us to a tee because of our fear of the inevitable, i.e., death. The term 'industry' gives away what it is all about. This industry banks on us falling sick and handing them all our hard-earned savings from all of our working life. It doesn't work in their favour to have healthy people who don't get sick often or postpone illness. It simply is a conflict of interest for them.

It is common knowledge, or at least it should be, that lifestyle choices play a role in lifestyle diseases like heart, lung and kidney conditions, cancers of all kinds, diabetes, etc. Most of these diseases don't happen overnight but build up over a period of time. It makes business sense to the so-called 'healthcare' industry that we lead a poor lifestyle. So, they are never genuinely keen on preventive approaches.

Nothing groundbreaking here. We all know this; it's just that we don't care.

In October 2021, Merck & Co., the pharmaceutical company that was the first to make smallpox vaccines commercially available in the US, announced that their experimental COVID pills halve the chances of hospitalization and death. Ironically, this led to a slump in shares of COVID vaccine makers.

Now you would think that is expected when you have a newer potential treatment. But is it? The scientific world knew for over six months of something else that had similar results.

A study[1] published in the *British Journal of Sports Medicine* in April 2021, conducted at Kaiser Permanente Southern California, US, looked at all COVID-19 positive cases they saw from 1 January 2020 to 21 October 2020, i.e., 48,440 adult patients. Researchers were interested in the physical activity of these people for the previous 2 years, i.e., from March 2018 to March 2020. They had three categories: consistently inactive (0–10 minutes per week), some activity (11–149 minutes per week) and consistently active (over 150 minutes per week).

Those who had been consistently inactive, basically the slobs who didn't even clock ten minutes of physical activity or exercise in a week, had a 2.26 times greater risk of hospitalization, 1.73 times greater risk of ICU admission and 2.49 greater risk of death due to COVID-19 than those who were active for 150 minutes in a week.

You would have thought that all governments, policymakers, hospitals and doctors would have been yelling about this from the rooftops. The problem is that being active and doing exercises doesn't really make any money for the big industries out there. That leads to lack of motivation.

Instead of promoting physical activity, sporting facilities were the last ones to be opened up. Interestingly, some countries did build an allowance of 'daily exercise' into their guidelines for the periods of lockdown. For example, in the UK, it was possible to leave your home for up to 60 minutes to 'exercise'. Unfortunately, the government missed a trick by not actually providing any guidance as to what people should be doing as part of this 'exercise'. When schools were opening up after almost 2 years, there were instructions from governments to not let students meet up for sporting activities.

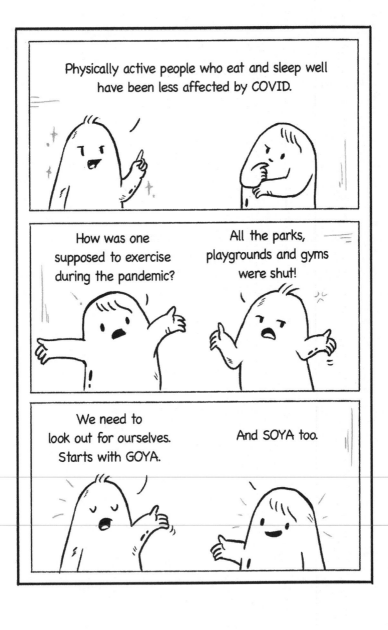

If we don't take responsibility for ourselves and our loved ones, it suits everyone else in this capitalistic world to take us for a ride, for as long as we let them. Unfortunately, most of us think that nothing will happen to us but only to people around us. The problem is that nothing goes wrong till it does, and when it does, it is too late and you can do nothing about it.

There is a good reason why physical activity hasn't really caught on at a mass level even after us being aware for almost seven decades now, and it makes sense that it annoys experts like Prof. Panteleimon (Paddy) Ekkekakis who've been at it for decades. Prof. Ekkekakis will be mentioned a number of times throughout this book for a reason, as he is a distinguished academic at Iowa State University in the field of exercise psychology and behaviour. Importantly, he focuses on the pleasure (and sometimes displeasure) of exercise, movement and play. We need to get fun into play. When you see dogs and other animals playing with each other, they are not following any plan, schedule or routine. They are doing it for fun. When we look back through the generations, it was through physical work, play and games that our ancestors would exercise. In modern society, with all the different forms of entertainment, our attention is taken away from what is good for us. Instead of being active, we find ourselves sitting and staring at a screen watching trash TV or browsing through social media to live other people's lives.

Whereas, when there was no awareness of exercise and fitness, our ancestors were very active, whether they were hunter-gatherers or even farmers. This may have been enough to move more throughout the day when the physical demands of daily life were greater. But for us, there are too many conveniences removing the necessity for physical movement. The biggest difference here is the need to exercise. Our hunter-gatherer ancestors had to move to avoid being killed by predators as well as to seek out their own prey. To move was the essence and purpose of life. Modern society though, through the comforts of supermarkets and the ability to get all that we need to survive at the click of a button, has transformed us into sedentary beings. Unfortunately for us as a species, such developments have outpaced evolution, which means that we have not yet adapted to the environment in which we now live.

Life

It's life we give them here. Not a career.

That's a quote by Dustin Hoffman's character, Master Carvelle, in the Hollywood film *Boychoir.*[2] Sadly, most institutions in the world, including the best of them, don't appreciate this enough.

We have all studied biology in school and/or college to some extent or the other, whether as part of science in primary and middle school; as biology itself in high school or in greater depth at a medical college. It is an important subject because it is about life, although there is not enough taught about the fundamentals of this life. We have all been given one life, or at least the one we think we are sure about. All the rest are just assumptions based on our upbringing, cultures and beliefs.

Unfortunately, the way it's taught in elementary or more advanced levels is through a tunnel vision approach. Barely any school applies any of the knowledge practically. For most people, the purpose of studying is to pass and excel in examinations to get jobs with higher salaries. In the process, they sadly forget about the lessons that would hold them in good stead for life, no matter what the circumstances. They address physical aspects of the person, without appreciating the surrounding society and environment enough. Even physically, there is mention of the hardware, i.e., the body and the brain, but somehow, the mind, which is the software that gives each of us our identity, is missed out.

Mental health and the implications of what happens when things aren't perfect are barely touched upon, if at all. That's appalling when an extremely high percentage of schoolgoing children today have mental health issues unlike ever before. This needs to be introduced and discussed early on in life. Only when children are aware of the mind will they know what is healthy or unhealthy.

Then there is sleep. Starting from our home and school, the belief that sleep is for the lazy is deeply ingrained in our minds. We are reminded time and again that if we need to get anywhere in life, be it in academics or sports, we need to sacrifice sleep to get more hours in the day to master things we want to excel in. Even if the importance of sleep, both in terms of quality and quantity, is touched upon, it is not with any seriousness. We just do not understand the implications of poor sleep.

Nutrition has been the one subject that has been taught the most but, for ages, it was based on the wrong information with the focus on high carbohydrates and proteins and fats being treated like the enemy. To make matters worse, given school timings, it simply doesn't make sense that for the most formative years, most children end up eating breakfast and lunch out of their tiffin boxes. Midday meals are crucial in schools, particularly with underprivileged children, but for the rest of the time, we need to think really hard about healthy food.

Fortunately, over the last two decades, there has been an increasing discussion about the role of physical activity, exercises and sports in overall health. Now you would have thought that everyone would be up and about, but as we all know, that's not the case.

A 2002 *New York Times* article titled, '5 Decades of Warnings Fail to Get Americans Moving' quoted a 1957 *US News & World Report.*[3]

> 'There is deep concern in high places over the fitness of American youth,' the magazine's report began. 'Parents are being warned that their children -- taken to school in buses, chauffeured to activities, freed from muscle-building chores and entertained in front of TV sets -- are getting soft and flabby.'

Seven decades later, the situation is no better. What needs to change is our messaging. Leave alone seven decades, we've known from the Ramayana and the Mahabharata era that the mind and body need to be fit. For the desired result of getting people to move more, we can't be using terms like warning and prescription. We need to change our narrative. It needs to be for fun. The *New York Times* article mentioned above was tweeted[4] by Prof. Ekkekakis, who has been at the forefront of trying to eradicate the physical inactivity pandemic.

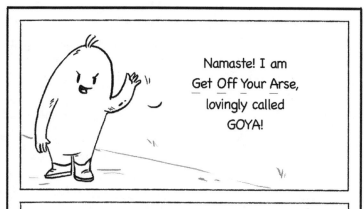

Namaste! I am Get Off Your Arse, lovingly called GOYA!

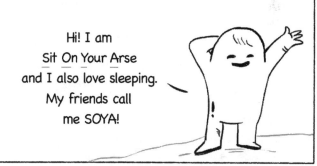

Hi! I am Sit On Your Arse and I also love sleeping. My friends call me SOYA!

Either get offended by us or get off your cute, royal backside and be a better you.

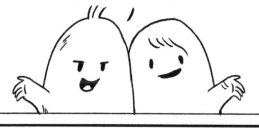

This pandemic is far greater and wide-reaching than the COVID pandemic, but no vaccine is ever going to get us out of it.

In response to Prof. Ekkekakis' tweet, Scott Douglas, a runner, author, health journalist and contributing writer for *Runner's World*, tweeted:[5]

> 'Warnings.' Always so effective in changing long-term behaviour. Jonathan Beverly, editor-in-Chief, Podium Runner at Outside, Inc. told me about a great framework used in his father's evangelical work. Instead of saying, 'You're living wrong, here's what you should be doing . . .' say, 'Here's how I live, and here's how great it is.'[6]

If only schools the world over had followed Jonathan's dad's formula and teachers led by example. Even if schools and colleges touch or focus on any of the four pillars of health mentioned above, i.e., physical activity, mental health, sleep and nutrition, they are almost definitely not addressing all four, and for sure, are not making connections between them. How can all these institutions miss out on this basic connection that is relevant to all of us for life?

Something very similar happens in medical colleges. As excited as medical students are to rid people of their sufferings, for the first 2 years, they often end up seeing no patients. The subjects taught in the first 2 years are called basic sciences as they lay the foundation for medicine. They may be termed 'basic sciences', but they are far from basic. In fact, they are so complex that the simple and most important elements of these subjects are forgotten.

During this period, the very first patient that medical students see is a cadaver—a dead body—through which an immense amount is learnt about the structures in the body. But unlike you and me, this body doesn't move, think, feel, eat or sleep. When medical students eventually start seeing patients who are alive and can move, think, feel, eat and sleep, they have a lot more subjects to stay abreast of. Somehow, they don't see the difference between the cadaver and the patients they see throughout their lives. They subconsciously end up addressing them in the same way—dead—rather than as human beings who are alive and have feelings.

Patch yourself

> *Doctors are (women and) men who prescribe medicines of which they know little, to cure diseases of which they know less, in human beings of whom they know nothing.*
>
> —Voltaire[7]

It was in 1998 that the popular Hollywood film, *Patch Adams*,[8] starring Robin Williams was released. It wasn't just a comedy, but the actual story of Dr Adams, who then, and even today, wants to change the way the healthcare system functions. As is often the case, the film didn't do justice to what the real Dr Adams, MD, is all about. The film picked up on how eccentric Patch was before he became Dr Adams, and how he ran the first 'silly hospital' in history but missed out on addressing other important points. Below, we present to you the real person who is a lot more interesting and passionate than the character showcased in the film and who continues to carry on with his mission of making this world a better place.

At the age of eighteen, before Adams was a medical student, he was hospitalized three times because he wanted to kill himself. He didn't want to live in a world full of violence and injustice. During the third hospitalization, he had a realization. 'You don't have to kill yourself, (when) you can make revolution.' He then decided to dedicate his life to a revolution called loving.[9]

> How can I, in every single waking moment, be an instrument for peace, justice and care? So, I decided that it was quite an easy decision. I would be happy, disgustingly happy, every single second of my life. I very quickly realized that it was six qualities: Happy, Funny, Loving, Cooperative, Creative & Thoughtful.
>
> And I decided to do it because my mother gave me self-esteem. All I had to do was to do it. I had been clownish before. I noticed when I was clowning, that clowning was a trick to get love close. So, I have clowned every day for 49 years (now 60 years).[10]

Some would pass this off as eccentric behaviour but it might surprise some of you that in a recent book published on the last day of 2019, *The Joy of Movement: How Exercise Helps Us Find Happiness, Hope, Connection, and Courage*, Dr Kelly McGonigal, a health psychologist and lecturer at Stanford University, who has taught dance, yoga and group exercise in the San Francisco Bay Area since 2000, concludes that 'movement offers us pleasure, identity, belonging and hope. It puts us in places that are good for us, whether that's outdoors in nature, in an environment that challenges us, or with a supportive community. It allows us to redefine ourselves and re-imagine what is possible. It makes social connection easier and self-transcendence possible'.[11]

Prof. Ekkekakis is also of the same opinion that we need to think more about psychology instead of exercise if we want more and more people to be active for life.[12] The pleasure of doing sports and exercise is more important than health. It does get annoying when massive events like the Olympics, time and again, become missed opportunities to change the health of the world.[13] The best of us start questioning ourselves if it's time to throw in the towel. It is only when we begin to consider the factors of motivation, resilience and other aspects of psychology that we will make real progress in getting people active for life.

Dr Adams goes on to say, 'Health and healthcare are a human right for all people. I entered medical school in 1967 to use it as a vehicle for social change.'[14] That's exactly what we think too. Always consider not just physical but mental health too and the positive impact that can be made in society. We all need to play our part to make that change happen, as we are all members of society. It is too much of a task to expect only doctors and other healthcare professionals to change. In any case, if we don't make ourselves more aware and take care of ourselves to the best of our abilities, what right do we have to expect strangers to do it for us?

Dr Adams rightly says something about his own team, and we would say the same about the best doctors and healthcare workers out there even today, who are an endangered species. 'We can promise care, but we can never promise cure. We need the right to make a mistake.'[15] We are humans after all.

For that care, we need to know our patients. The first interview and consultation with an adult patient for Dr Adams is at least 3–4 hours long. He wants to understand them well. Treat them like human beings, as people, not just bodies. In a country like India, 3–4 hours for the first consultation would be extremely difficult, especially if we are to follow Dr Adams' model of not charging any fee, something he has done for the last 50 years. As a matter of fact, throughout his life, Dr Adams has paid to be a doctor.

In his first 12 years of practice, Dr Adams found that less than 3 per cent of the population he saw had any self-esteem, less than 5 per cent had any idea of what day-to-day vitality for life was about. Shocking numbers.

> The normal adult didn't like themselves, didn't like their marriage, and didn't like their job. That wasn't why they came to a doctor.[16]

That still holds true. Rajat has been seeing a similar pattern over his two plus decades of medical practice, first in the UK (London) and then in India (Bengaluru and Delhi), becoming a friend to most of his patients. And it has nothing to do with education, religion, gender, age or whichever corner of the world they come from. It is the same everywhere. For some reason, as humans, we have lost our way when it comes to a passion for life, which is now manifesting as poor physical and mental health.

Dr Adams adds, 'Practically no one was proactive about their health. That's why, from the beginning, we integrated Medicine with performing arts and crafts, agriculture, nature, education, recreation and social service. In a way, we used their disease as a gimmick to get them into a university of human culture. We were teaching love, joy, humour, passion, hope, wonder, curiosity, creativity, intimacy, shared efforts with people. We've been the only hospital to integrate all the healing arts. When we started, it was against the law. Our law is: what do the patients need? So, from the very beginning, everything you have ever heard of as complementary care, we have been involved in.'[17]

Dr Adams has been a whole system thinker. He wanted to create a hospital that addressed every single problem of healthcare delivery in one model. Through this book and project, we are trying to do the same but in a slightly different manner. We want to democratize medicine. As doctors, therapists and healthcare professionals, we need to take ourselves a little less seriously (yes, you read that right) and not be insecure about sharing our knowledge. It is also going to be important for professionals to drop their egos and appreciate the value of all those who work to improve health. This means doctors and other medical professionals must see the importance of complementary and alternative therapies in treating patients.

This is for all of us to ponder over. How can healthcare possibly only belong to folks who have random letters of the alphabet written after their names, wear white coats, have a tube of some sort around their necks and carry a title in front of their names for a profession which is no longer noble, and yet want their patients to be patient while they practise on them? Why should there be any distinction? Let's consider this. A plumber is an expert in the maintenance of drainage systems for homes, where we all spend most of our lifetimes. Yet, society considers them lowly as compared to cardiovascular surgeons, even though they both do similar jobs.

As Dr Adams says, 'All over the world, physicians are rude. There is a hierarchy, all over the world. There is deep sadness that you don't have enough time with patients.' 90 per cent of students and staff in his medical school were rude and arrogant. 'My mother taught me never (to be rude). That was about the worst thing a human could be. I couldn't believe how everyone was silent about it.' [18]

On graduating from Virginia Commonwealth University Medical School in 1971, Dr Adams, along with twenty of his friends, three of whom were doctors, started Gesundheit Institute in a large six-bedroom house. As Dr Adams mentions in his 2012 TEDx Talk in the Netherlands,[19] it was a hospital, just of a different kind, open 24 hours a day. They created an environment for the hospital which would be the same as Dr Adams decided for himself: happy, funny, loving, cooperative, creative and thoughtful. Again, these were the only six qualities that he expected his permanent staff to have. Those were the only degrees and qualifications he was looking for, and they mattered to him more than any piece of paper.

> 'They had 500 to 1000 people each month with five to fifty overnight guests a night. Everything was free—all the care and all the medicine—if need be.' As Dr Adams states in his book *Gesundheit*, 'It was an experiment in holistic medical care based on the belief that one cannot separate the health of the individual from the health of the family, the community and the world.'[20] It was a pilot project that lasted 12 years.
>
> One of the most important tenets of our philosophy is that health is based on happiness, from hugging and clowning around, to finding joy in family and friends. Satisfaction in work, ecstasy in nature and the arts. For us, healing is not only prescribing medicine and therapies, but working together, and sharing in the spirit of joy and

cooperation. Much more than simply a medical centre, Gesundheit facility will be a microcosm of life, integrating medical care with farming, arts and crafts, performing arts, education, nature, recreation, friendship, and fun. Yes, we want the world to change.[21]

Hospitals aren't happy places. They don't have happy people. When patients leave a hospital with improved health, it should be celebrated. This is starting to happen with some cancer treatments, but it does not happen enough.

The hierarchy that one sees in hospitals the world over is mastered in medical colleges. Hierarchy gives power to the people at the top, and as we all know, power corrupts. Most doctors become rude for no rhyme or reason, not respecting those who they had taken an oath to serve.

If only medical colleges taught compassion as an embedded course or in any other form at all. According to Dr Adams, 'Practice of Medicine is practice of compassion with whatever humble tools and knowledge that you have to help another person.'[22] We all need to start with having compassion for ourselves, being our best friends, before expecting any stranger called doctor to treat us that way. More than treating them like demigods, take care of the temple within.

Whether you are from the healthcare fraternity or not, you might think that compassion and empathy are already an integral part of the healthcare world since we are dealing with human beings and not machines. But is it? Research studies in this area, performed over two decades, have been done in countries around the world, across different cultures, like Peru,[23] Pakistan,[24] Malaysia,[25] Turkey,[26] China,[27] US,[28] Iran,[29] Portugal,[30] Syria[31] and India,[32] and have found something alarming. Compassion and empathy are usually higher among first year undergraduate medical students as compared to students from other streams, with women being more empathetic. Shockingly, as time passes by, when medical students move from basic science (the first 2 years when no patients are seen) to the clinical phase, there is a progressive and rapid decline in their empathy levels. Yet, this is the time when they first begin to meet real patients!

Going by this, you would almost know what to expect next. Research studies have also demonstrated that in the postgraduate medical stream, students tend to have more compassion and empathy as compared to those in surgical and technical specialities. There is a suggestion that starting clinical exposure earlier might help. But that could also possibly backfire and whatever empathy there may be, might just wane sooner.

It is almost like the curse Parashurama gave to Karna in the Mahabharat.[33] Parashurama only took in Brahmins[34] as his students. Karna, aware of that, lied to Parashurama, presenting himself as a Brahmin. Karna worked hard, improved at a rapid pace, and easily became the best student Parashurama had ever trained.

One day, after training, when Parashurama was tired and wanted to rest, Karna offered his lap to his guru. While Parashurama slept, a scorpion bit Karna on his thigh. Karna was bleeding and in extreme pain, but he still didn't flinch a muscle as that would have disturbed his guru. When Parashurama got up and saw the blood, rather than being thankful, he was furious. He immediately knew that Karna wasn't a Brahmin as a Brahmin wouldn't have stayed quiet with all that pain. He cursed Karna for having lied to him and said that during the most crucial battle of Karna's life, he would forget the most important lessons taught to him. As it turned out, when Karna needed to use the brahmastra to save his life, the most powerful weapon in his arsenal, he just couldn't remember how to, and that led to his death.

Doctors often face the same curse as Karna. They can forget the meaning of 'healthcare' and be empty of compassion when it is most needed. Yes, there are always exceptions, but that isn't the rule. Unfortunately, with the pressures of modern medicine, the exceptions are becoming rarer. This has become even more evident during the COVID-19 pandemic, when many people have not been seen by a doctor face to face for more than 2 years. Doctors have been forced to see images on a screen, rather than real patients, which has led to severe consequences in some circumstances.

The problem with humans is that we don't recognize what we don't know. We need to be humble enough to listen and change, which is not an easy ask. This is even more important for medical professionals, who need to be humble to admit they don't know and are not scared to contact other people who might be able to help. This can only happen when there are suitable role models, like Dr Adams himself.

All those in the healthcare industry need to have some humility to say that we don't know it all and that we are keen to learn more and become better.

It needs to be more like Councillor Hamann from *The Matrix Reloaded*.

> *There is so much in this world that I do not understand. I have absolutely no idea how it (water recycling machine) works. But I do understand the reason for it to work.*[35]

To address this problem, about a decade and a half ago, Dr Adams was instrumental in starting the world's first medical curriculum on 'Compassion in Healthcare' in partnership with Bolaroja Clown Doctors of Peru and Cayetano Heredia Medical School, a private non-profit university located in Lima, Peru.

If someone is not compassionate to themselves, how are they expected to be compassionate to others? Hence, we suggest the same for *MoveMint Medicine* in medical colleges across the world. We invite all and any colleges out there to contact us directly at an institutional level. We are even willing to connect with students directly. Again, why should compassion and knowing more about yourself be limited to medical colleges alone? We are keen to empower all students in schools and colleges of all kinds with knowledge to lead a better and happy life and not only to pass examinations and get high grades. All employees working in the private or public sector; all housewives and the elderly should also know better. It is not only your right but a duty to yourself. We'll make sure that it is fun and practical.

Together, we need to get rid of all the barriers to make change happen, one baby step at a time. We all need to remember that throughout history, the majority has always been led by the minority. Let us together be those pathfinders.

We simply can't outsource our health to doctors. We should all 'Move and Bee' for the joy of it. In any case, to Dr Adams, the health of the caregiver is as important as the health of the patients. Only if you can take care of yourself and are in a good physical and mental state, will you possibly be of any help to anyone else.

People will forget what you said, people will forget what you did, but people will never forget how you made them feel.
— Maya Angelou[36]

For that same reason, we urge all our doctors and healthcare colleagues to leave their ego aside and get on with this wonderful *MoveMint Medicine* journey, for your sake and for all those you care about, your loved ones and your patients. Let us begin to 'patch' up the broken healthcare system and heal the institutions that were set up to heal us.

2

The Three Musketeers (Don't 'Dis' Them)

On the evening of 15 October 2019, Rajat held his mother's head in his lap for over 8 hours. Nothing seemed structurally wrong with the three vital hardware required for life—lungs, heart and the brain. It was just that none of them were working. They had got permanently corrupted and shut down. She was dead. There is no polite way to put it. That spark called life was missing. Rajat simply couldn't understand why he, with all his medical knowledge in different fields and over two decades of experience, was not able to bring her back.

In hindsight, he appreciates that he was lucky to at least hold her, even if it was after she had passed away. The COVID era has challenged humanity itself where people didn't get to see, leave alone touch, their loved ones before they were cremated or buried.

Lungs. Heart. Brain. These three musketeers are the vital hardware for life. They work in sync to keep you alive, every second and minute of the day. The better doctors and healthcare professionals might have spoken to you about them, but barely anyone discusses the software that keeps you

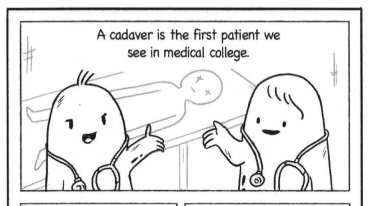

A cadaver is the first patient we see in medical college.

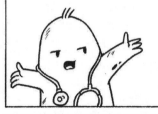

And the dead teach the living a lot.

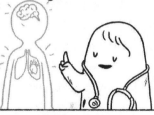

We learn about vital organs like the heart, the lungs and the brain.

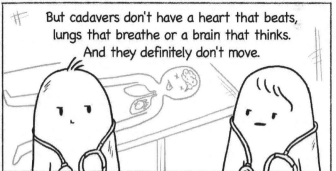

But cadavers don't have a heart that beats, lungs that breathe or a brain that thinks. And they definitely don't move.

alive. Breathing, without which you wouldn't come into this world and move on to the next level; heartbeat which makes blood flow throughout the body, and finally, the mind which is far beyond the brain. If that spark of life is missing, all that hardware is of no use.

Dys-function Precedes Dis-ease

If you want to understand a human body, you do need to understand its functions simultaneously. If only we ourselves, as well as medical professionals, could recognize and address 'dys-function' before 'dis-ease', the world would be a healthier place. Sadly, the traditional Western medicine approach doesn't look at things like that. They don't go beyond the body, if at all. Usually, they have a very microscopic view, which does not even involve looking at the whole human body, but just a diseased or injured body part. We need to acknowledge that it's not our knee that has pain, or the lung that has tuberculosis, or a heart that has an attack, or the brain that has a stroke, or cancer of a certain body part. Those are just symptoms, nameplates that our doctor colleagues brand you with.

You can know the name of a bird in all the languages of the world, but when you're finished, you'll know absolutely nothing whatsoever about the bird . . . So let's look at the bird and see what it's doing—that's what counts.

—Prof. Richard Feynman[1]

You are a lot more than that body part and there is a lot more to you than that moment of time. If you don't respect and value that, how do you expect anyone else to do that? As Prof. Feynman said, it is very important for you to know yourself better and why something ails you.

Don't 'Dis' It

We need to learn how to get rid of the 'dys' and the 'dis', to be able to function with ease. And to function with ease, the whole of you and all your past experience are needed. You need to think about your physical and mental self, as well as your diet and sleep. You need to do *MoveMint*. It is something all animals know and practise without the need to think, probably because they have no option. It is just that comfortable humans forget about it all since we are 'educated'. It is probably because we lose touch with our own selves, the need for survival and the environment around us. Again, we are not trying to make you doctors, but are trying to make you more aware of yourself, the entity that you are a CEO of. You! If you don't take ownership of your own self, who else will?

The ethical debate about when a growing human develops a mind and thoughts is an age-old one. However, one thing is clear—we moved to be born, first as a sperm and an ovum. Then we moved as a foetus; had the most balanced nutrition and slept in the security of our mother's womb before finally moving into this world as a newborn child. But was it at a constant pace throughout? Had we, as a foetus continued to grow for the whole nine months at the same rate that we were growing at 5–6 weeks in the womb, you and I would have been 1.5 tonnes (i.e., 1500 kg) at birth.[2] A similar thing happened with the birth of the universe, if we are to go by the 'big bang', the widely accepted theory of the beginning of everything that exists as we know and don't know, which supposedly happened 13.8 billion years ago. At the very beginning, very similar to the foetus, the universe expanded from an initial stage of high density (and temperature too). In the first picosecond, i.e., 1/1000,000,000,000 (one trillionth) of a second, no rules of physics applied.[3]

A picosecond is to one second what one second is to approximately 31,689 years.[4] Differently put, a trillion seconds is the number of seconds that all of us, say here in Delhi, will spend in a day. If only one of us just said the word 'second' it would be a trillionth of all the seconds lived in a day by all the residents, of the Indian capital.

Basically, it's a unit of time that is extremely difficult to comprehend. For that minuscule fraction of a second, the universe expanded at a mind-boggling speed. And then, the growth of expansion suddenly slowed down remarkably.

Had the universe carried on growing at that pace, it would have torn itself apart. As much as we have been told about how pace is constant, the rate of growth of a human and the birth of the universe will remind you that pace is never constant. At the right time, the pace needs to be increased and then reduced for optimal results. Tiny ripples that happened in the universe at that stage are believed to be the basis of all events that have ever happened, are happening now or will ever happen in the future. And no, we are not only talking about your love interests, how much money you'll make, Indian or even US politics. We, as a planet, are insignificant in the bigger scheme of things, but there are similarities to be found everywhere.[5]

It is important to appreciate that nature is pretty much the same, anywhere we see. Repercussions of messing around with it can be fatal. As the ripples of the 'big bang' have and will continue to determine all of the universe's future, so will messing around with the nature of human beings. But that's exactly what we have been doing for a while, at an insane pace in the last couple of decades.

From pretty much the turn of this century, as soon as humans are born, they are being introduced to smartphones and gadgets, as if they are born with these devices in their hand. Never mind 'smart', these technologies are dumbing the species that prides itself to be the smartest, and hence on top of the food chain. Yes, adaptation is the one characteristic that really makes us unique. It is just that we have adapted to a very sad and harmful lifestyle. Unfortunately, as a species, we have gravitated towards things that are bad for us and away from the things that are good for us. We simply aren't moving enough, not resting when we ought to, not eating what and when we should, while our mental health is royally messed up, all of them getting worse with each passing generation. And the fault lies not with the current generation but the ones before as they are trying to fix things based on what they've gone through, rather than thinking about what the future holds.

That's ironic because as much as there is more and more talk of exercise and physical activity publicized through the multiple channels of media that now exist, it is in an era when there is the least physical activity of all humankind. We need to get back to moving, a whole lot more. We need to connect with nature and sleep accordingly. We need to be eating what naturally works for us. And we need to value ourselves and be our best friend. Mental health needs to be given priority. No, ignoring it is not going to fix a thing as we are now sitting on a time bomb when we should be getting off our royal backsides and doing something about it proactively.

Breathe: Lungs

For breath is life, and if you breathe well, you will live long on earth.

—Sanskrit proverb

It's for this reason that 'pran' means 'life' as well as 'breath' in Hindi and Sanskrit. And it has nothing to do with philosophy, not that we shouldn't be aware of it. It is about science that somehow medical students aren't often reminded of after their initial 2 years in college. These doctors soon forget that the essence of breathing, if practised incorrectly, can be the very cause of dysfunction and disease.

When we enter this world, if we are not already crying, the attending nurse or doctor pats our back to make us bawl. And with that, our life starts. Crying! We carry on the tradition of crying throughout our lives whether we internalize it or showcase it to the world externally. We forget what the main purpose of that cry initially was. It wasn't about sadness, even though throughout life that's what it gets associated with. The cry was to forcefully clear the airways. With that, we exhale. This would be followed by inhalation of fresh air. If we didn't first empty out, there would have been no space for any air to come in. And this out–in should apply to all that we do in life.

The next breath the society pays attention to happens to be the last one. 'So-and-so took his or her last breath at a certain time.' The vital role breathing plays throughout life is totally undermined. It is not only important for a long life, but also for leading a quality life. We all somehow take breathing for granted. Given how important breathing is for life, why are we never taught how to breathe properly? Maybe, we don't need to be taught, but we definitely should be repeatedly reminded and be reminding others to mindfully breathe, as we simply can't overdo it. If you are not breathing properly, your body will not function properly and hence, it will be forced into adapting ways to try and keep you alive.

Although as a newborn, we breathe naturally without conscious thought or effort, from that day forward, breathing becomes less and less natural. If it is important for life, it should make sense that it is important for everything else during that life too. So, when was the last time your doctor told you to breathe? They are busy giving you an exotic name tag for the problem you have gone to them for, almost boasting about how intelligent they are.

When adults try to run, the first complaint or feedback is that they get breathless with a few minutes of running. Step back and think about it. When you have taken breathing for granted while lying down, sitting or standing, how do you expect it to miraculously be in sync with your running and not make you breathless? Just think again.

What does breathing do? The oxygen-loaded inhaled air, passing through the nose and the windpipe, and gets into the lungs. In the lungs, it goes to the smallest units of the lungs called the alveoli. Here, the oxygen is offloaded by the inhaled air and gets into the blood, flowing in the blood pipes going back to the heart. At the same time, that blood from the heart releases carbon dioxide, which then mixes with the air, and is then exhaled out. Oxygen-rich blood now goes back to the heart, the central pump of the human body. From here, this oxygen-rich blood is sent throughout the body as oxygen plays a vital role for all kinds of functions in every cell of the body. And so, the cycle continues.

Bus and the Bus Stop

Imagine that breath you take in to be a bus loaded with oxygen. The two lungs are the bus stop. When we don't think much about breathing, the bus (breath) goes towards the bus stop (lungs), but barely stops there. Only a few oxygen molecules get a chance to get off and only a few carbon dioxide molecules get a chance to get on the bus.

A similar thing happens when one breathes fast and shallow while trying to run or while playing a sport, or even while having an anxiety attack. That bus (breath) speeds towards the bus stop (lungs) but, in a rush, barely stops there for a few milliseconds.

Both the above situations lead us to work suboptimally whether at work, school, home or while playing a sport. Why? Because you don't have an optimal amount of oxygen getting to the cellular level for optimal working. This would limit or slow down recovery from an injury or a disease. For lack of oxygen, we increase the frequency of buses (breaths) even more, but it makes the bus (breath) stop for an even shorter period at the bus stop (lungs), leading to higher need of oxygen. This vicious cycle goes on and then we have no idea what to do about our breathing. That's exactly the dilemma we find ourselves in while trying to run fast or during an asthmatic episode.

This seems like we are all doomed and there is no solution in sight. But there is, and it's a lot simpler than you would think.

This time, the bus (breath) heads towards the bus station (lungs) but is not in a rush. It's going gently. On getting to the bus stop (lungs), it stops there for all the oxygen molecules to get off and all the carbon dioxide to get on, and only then does it start moving again, slowly. This helps get enough oxygen into the blood headed towards the heart and from there being sent to the brain and the rest of the body. This simple act of slowing down the bus (breath) helps us function optimally.

That's why, this quote from the film *Shooter* makes a lot of sense. 'Slow is smooth. Smooth is fast.'[6] Or in running terms, if you want to run as fast as you can, slow down. This is why we have set you the task of concentrating on your breathing. If you start doing this regularly, it will eventually become second nature. There may be some situations where your breathing is not in tune. For example, when you are stressed, anxious, or even when you are running. But with the right amount of time and practice, breathing in these situations will also improve.

Therapeutic Relaxed Breathing

Pick a quiet room—it must be as quiet as you can make it. This is your me zone. If there are any distractions in the room, then remove them. There should be no TV, phone or other gadget that might suddenly make noise. Sit tall like a puppet having a string attached to the top of the head, with your shoulders and chest relaxed. If sitting tall is painful, sit or lie down in the position that is most comfortable. You need to focus on breathing out (exhaling) as only by emptying the lungs will they have optimal capacity to breathe in (inhale) fresh amounts of air. Reminding yourself to relax your body,

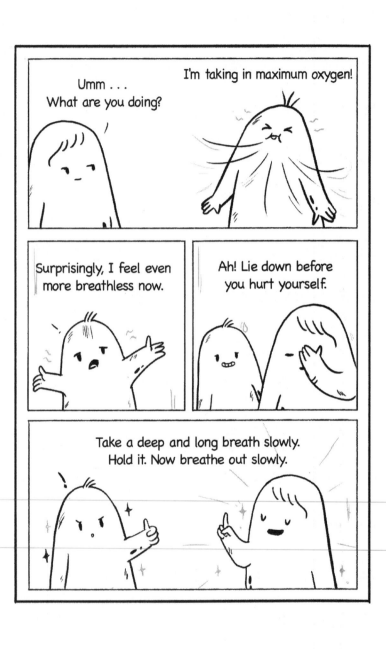

slowly and at a constant pace, exhale out over a count of seven. You could time yourself using a watch. This might seem like a long duration to start with, but you'll soon get used to it. Now inhale over a count of four. This will seem a lot easier as lungs tend to suck in air because of the air pressure difference created between lungs and the outside air during exhalation. For our purpose, we would suggest letting the ribs expand and rise each time you breathe in. The diaphragm will anyway do what it is supposed to do. Repeat it five times.

Once you've got the hang of breathing pace, you need to move on to the next level. You should now do the above breathing technique with your eyes closed. In addition to that, to distract yourself from the pain in your body and in life, we want you to do a reverse count, i.e., count from seven to zero while exhaling and count from four to zero while inhaling.

In the next level, once you are fully comfortable with breathing pace, do a reverse count from fifty-five to zero for the whole exercise. Over time, you can do it over 111 seconds, 222 seconds, 333 seconds and 555 seconds. To be fully involved in this activity, you might want to do a reverse count of odd numbers, divisible by three, seven, eleven, etc. Again, the intent is to get you distracted from all that life has thrown at you.

If you are finding it difficult to maintain focus, you should use your imagination to take you somewhere that helps you to stay in tune with your breathing. You may wish to imagine the waves of the sea going in and out, or the repetitive motion of a swing or the hand of a pendulum clock. Being in tune with this imagery will help to keep focus and maintain rhythm with your breathing. Your racing mind will try to take you away from this relaxing and necessary practice, so you may need to play with different imagery techniques to help you.

Therapeutic Relaxed Breathing

This is how we can progress over time with our breathing:

Level 1: In a quiet room and in a tall posture, exhale for over 7 seconds and inhale for over 4 seconds. Repeat this five times.
Level 2: Close your eyes, exhale for over 7 seconds and inhale for over 4 seconds. Repeat this five times.
Level 3: Repeat level 2 but count from fifty-five to 0 for the whole exercise.
Levels 4–7: Repeat level 2, but count from 111 to 0, 222 to 0, 333 to 0 and 555 to 0.

Heartbeat

We all know that the heartbeat is important, but the heart is only beating to pump oxygenated blood throughout the body for all vital functions to be carried out at cellular levels. Beating without any blood or oxygen would serve no purpose whatsoever. That oxygenated blood, or oxygen-rich blood is totally dependent on your breathing. Coaches, sportspeople and runners amongst readers should then wonder why is it that the latest gadgets are measuring heartbeats and pulse to help with your performance but not your breathing? Rajat always tells runners or wannabe runners being mentored by him to focus on their breathing and to run at the pace of their breath and not breathe at the pace of their running.

The heart can be considered the most important organ of the human body. Indeed, we are all aware of the consequences if the heart stops beating for an extended period of time. Even if it stops for a short duration, the consequences can be devastating and life-changing.

With all that being said, despite all of the intricate complexities, the heart is simply a mechanical pump. Its one and only job is to pump blood in two directions: to the lungs, so that the blood can be filled with oxygen, and the other way, to the rest of the body, where the blood containing oxygen can be supplied to organs and tissues. For this to happen, there are two sides of the heart which correspond to the two directions in which the blood needs to flow. These sides are further split into chambers, so there are four chambers in total. The two top chambers (known as atria) receive the blood (from the body and lungs respectively), whilst the two bottom chambers (known as ventricles) collect the blood before it is squeezed out. Blood is allowed to flow from the top to the bottom chambers, with the opening of special valves. There are pipes (vessels) that carry the blood into the heart and then out of the heart in the correct direction, with the aorta (main vessel leading to the rest of the body) being able to withstand the incredible pressure needed to transport the blood over incredible distances. As an analogy, you can imagine that the heart is like the 'boiler' of a central heating system in a house. If any of the pipes get blocked, or worse, burst, or if the pump fails, there will be a major problem requiring immediate attention.

Like the muscles in our limbs (skeletal muscles), the heart is itself a muscle, which when contracted, squeezes out blood with tremendous force. Imagine taking a wet dishcloth and squeezing it to get all of the water out—that is exactly what the heart does with every single beat. Unlike our skeletal muscle, the heart never tires, unless there is a problem, which we will go on to talk about subsequently. Your heart beats approximately 1,00,000 times per day, 35 million times per year and 2.5 billion times across your lifetime. All this happens without you having to think about it once! For it to be able to perform like this, the heart needs its own blood supply. It is one of the major pipes of this supply system that can often get narrow or blocked, which is known as coronary artery disease. Common interventions can include removing the blockage and also putting a 'stent' in place to open the pipe and prevent it from being blocked. Further still, heart surgeons can perform bypasses to connect the parts of the pipe together that are not blocked, literally bypassing the blockage.

These interventions can be very successful and allow people to return to their 'normal' lives. Darren remembers that his grandfather had a triple heart bypass when he was middle-aged but lived until his nineties. Unfortunately, there is a reason that these pipes get blocked and if the issues are not addressed, there can be recurring and often more devastating consequences. The combination of a poor diet and lack of physical activity causes the pipes to narrow, become stiffer (not letting as much blood through) and ultimately, to get blocked.

Your heartbeat is controlled by what is known as the autonomic (automatic) nervous system. Although your heart knows how and when to beat, you can still have some control over it, such as through the breathing exercises above, which will help slow heartbeat down. There is a highly controlled electrical network which controls your heartbeat, which can go wrong in certain medical conditions. Fortunately for us, we can also use electricity to get the heart beating again if it stops. This is what we know as a defibrillator, which literally 'shocks' the heart into beating properly again.

In the age of connected smart devices, we all seem to want to measure our heart rate, either when we rest or during exercise. Although heart rate has been used to measure the intensity of exercise for decades, without knowing it, we are much better at monitoring how intense the exercise actually is. We should all pay more attention to how our body feels, being in tune with breathing as the basics of movement, rather than relying on a number that appears on our watch or app.

Let's step back again. Where is it that the pair of lungs and the heart reside? It's called a ribcage. These ribs, twelve of them, are connected at the back to twelve bones of the spine, stacked on top of each other and are collectively called the thoracic vertebrae. There are seven bones in the neck called the cervical vertebrae that are further stacked on top of them. The seven neck bones and the twelve upper and middle backbones are further stacked on five lower backbones called the lumbar vertebrae. These twenty-four bones of the spine have to have both agility and stability for good health.

Simply put, there are twenty-four bones sitting on top of each other from your belt level till the skull at the top. Ribs are attached to roughly the middle half of them.

All the ribs, in the ribcage at the front, are connected to a 'tie'-like bone called the sternum. At the back, as mentioned above, they are attached to the twelve thoracic vertebrae of the upper and middle back. Effectively, your two lungs and the heart reside in this cage. Each of these ribs, on both the left

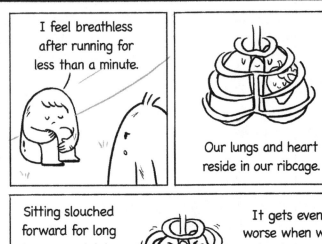

I feel breathless after running for less than a minute.

Our lungs and heart reside in our ribcage.

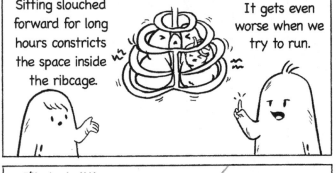

Sitting slouched forward for long hours constricts the space inside the ribcage.

It gets even worse when we try to run.

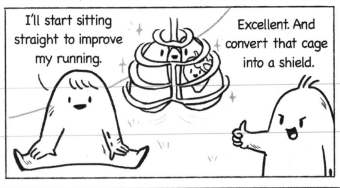

I'll start sitting straight to improve my running.

Excellent. And convert that cage into a shield.

and the right sides of the body, are like a bucket handle. Think of twelve bucket handles stacked on top of each other on both sides. When we take a long breath in, all these bucket handles move up, increasing the volume of that ribcage. When we exhale, all these bucket handles collapse on top of each other, reducing the volume of the ribcage. It is muscles that control the movement of all of these bones, in a highly coordinated fashion to make the process as efficient as possible. Now this happens whether you are doing diaphragmatic (belly) breathing or not. Think of the amount of coordination that is needed for just a single breath in and a single breath out.

The basic posture of humans today is extremely poor and does not support and facilitate efficient breathing. As we have said before, courtesy of the advancements in technology, more so in the last two decades, every child seems to be born with a smartphone attached to their hands. Very early on, children start slouching to get engrossed with that screen. Adults too are not immune to this. Think of the spine and that ribcage. When we slouch, that ribcage with twelve of its handles on both sides collapses down, restricting upward movement, reducing the extent to which they can increase the volume inside. Soon, the range of motion of the ribs, in turn, limits the movement of the spine, becoming a permanent habit.

Why is this important to understand? This newly acquired posture doesn't let you move optimally, compromising all other bodily functions too. Think about it: your lungs and heart don't have the freedom to expand freely and feel constricted all the time. In fact, the muscles that help all of the bones to move try their very best to help overcome the poor posture, but soon get tired and affected themselves. If the heart, lungs and brain, the three musketeers vital for life, are not working optimally, how will the rest of your body be in good shape? No, you don't need to be a doctor or even a rocket scientist to figure this out.

Zoom out a little bit more and you'll now see the whole human body. When one visits an orthopaedic doctor whether in their clinic or in the hospital setting, almost always, there is a skeleton hanging in the reception area. Subconsciously, the message that registers is that you are just that—a bag full of bones—somehow put together. The skeleton is placed there with the intention of either explaining to you what may be going on with you, or it is thought to be an appropriate part of the interior design for such a facility. The skeleton is important, but everything that surrounds the skeleton is just as important too. Yet, it is not shown. What about your psychological well-being, and eating and sleeping habits?

There is that skull which might scare you, but as mentioned earlier, the skull is merely smiling back at you. Then there is the rest of the skeleton with all its bones hanging. Bones in these artificial skeletons are held together by wires, nuts and bolts. Skeletons within all of us living beings, on the other hand, are held together by muscles, tendons and ligaments, and we possess the capacity to think and feel, all of which is almost always forgotten about. It's yet again these muscles, tendons and ligaments that get us moving. And that's why they become crucial to our good health. But where is it that muscles and bones get instructions to get us moving? Because they can't move on their own.

It's the spine, starting as a brain along with the whole network of nerves, that is the chassis for this whole skeleton of ours. Audi's technology website sums it up really well. 'The sporty character of all Audi models is essentially rooted in their chassis. Sophisticated yet lightweight suspension and steering systems, powerful brakes and highly intelligent electronics together make for a fascinating driving experience.'[7] That's what we want all of you to think of yourselves as—the most sophisticated machinery ever created. Let's then not treat ourselves like trash. Most of us wouldn't do that to our Audis. And those who do, definitely don't deserve that Audi.

As the Audi's chassis has 'highly intelligent electronics', so does the human spine. The brain, stationed in the top chamber of the skeleton called the skull, continues as the spinal cord in the spine. As mentioned earlier, from the base of the skull, till the level where we would wrap a belt around our waist, there are twenty-four vertebral bones that are stacked on top of each other from the belt level. Each of these vertebrae are awkwardly designed. They are not a cube or a cylinder but designed in such a way that they fit well like pieces of a jigsaw. All these bones have a hole in the centre through which the spinal cord passes with the spinal bones safeguarding it. At each of the twenty-four levels, there are nerves which branch out and supply electricity to different parts of the body. Imagine this like a telegraph signal or electricity trip box.

No, we weren't gifted Audi's (or as Darren prefers, BMWs!) and they didn't sponsor this book. Audi or any other car for that reason would be no good if we couldn't turn on the ignition and get moving. That's what the first breath and the first heartbeat are all about. But after that, every movement and function that the body does is triggered and supervised by the brain, the central processor unit. Then how dare we let anyone treat us like a bagful of bones or a piece of furniture alone? The onus is on us, and for that, we don't need any kind of fancy degrees. The interesting part is that the doctors and healthcare professionals who would agree with us are the ones who lead by example and preach *MoveMint Medicine* knowingly or unknowingly. As for those who disagree with us, we shouldn't really worry about them too much. Their ego is a bit too inflated to let anyone make any sense to them until their ego gets punctured and then they learn the hard way.

Once we overcome the initial barrier to get moving and decide to become our own best friend, it's game on. It's the brain sending a signal through the spinal cord that the muscles must get those bones and joints to move.

Down the line, we make the right choices for nutrition and sleep too.

But why do we decide to do that or not?

Before we talk further about the body, we first need to understand more about the mind. Why do we think what we think and why do we do what we do? Once we understand this, dealing with our own health and disease will be a lot easier.

Smile

It goes back to something fundamental. As much as we are all scared of the skeleton that we may have seen in the doctor's consultation room, especially the skull, reinforced repeatedly by Hollywood and Bollywood films alike, there is one thing that we all miss to appreciate. If you look at the skull, it is smiling, proudly showcasing the thirty-two teeth, or whatever is left of them, in all their glory. Similarly, if you were to look at the scan of an unborn baby, you will notice it smiling back at you. So what if those glorious teeth are missing at this stage. The amazing 3D and 4D scans that are now available during pregnancy give incredible resolutions of the baby in the womb—maybe the baby is so happy because it is getting everything it needs in its perfect environment.

From the time before our birth to the time after our death, the skeleton is smiling. Then what happens while we are alive? Why are we all frowning and struggling to smile? It is because we are covered by layers and layers. Funny then that we need muscles to smile when deep inside, below all those layers of skin, fascia and muscles, by default, we are smiling. Even so, when we smile, tensing all those muscles of the face, the muscles over the rest of the body relax. Smiling has a calming effect, whether forced or real. Try that right now. Smile. From ear to ear. Go for it. And now practise that from year to year. Even though practice doesn't make perfect, it does make it permanent. Even that imperfect smile, if there is anything like that, is far better than a frown. Even better, it is infectious, and the other person looking at you will genuinely smile back.

Get on with this experiment today itself. Take time to smile at everyone (when safe to do so!), known and unknown today. Keep a count of how many smiled back at you. Do this for a month, keeping a note of how you felt each day. It could be on a scale of ten. You'll notice that your happiness quotient will start improving. And that's an important component of *MoveMint Medicine*.

We have covered the mind right after this section but it is important to mention here that without the mind, all of the human body, being in as mint shape that it possibly could be, can't do a thing. In fact, in order for the physical body to be in the best shape it can be, the mind needs to be in good shape too. The saying 'healthy body, healthy mind' is true, but so is 'healthy mind, healthy body'. After all, if you do not have the right mindset, your sleep, physical activity and nutrition will not be optimal.

The healthcare fraternity just hasn't given the mind and mental health its due. Unfortunately, because of this, issues related to mental health and well-being are rapidly rising among all of us. We find it fascinating when our colleagues in this age have an epiphany as to how important a role the mind plays, whether it be in pain or any chronic disease. But then again, better late than never. Mental health is starting to become more recognized through public health campaigns, but there is still a long way to go. As individuals, we also have a role to play by acknowledging our own state of mental health and knowing how to be open to talk about it and to seek help when needed.

As the heart helps with heartbeats and the lungs with breathing, the brain is where the mind resides, and it thinks. It is crucial to our being, to us being human beings. After all, we are a sum total of all our experiences, what we make of them and how we react. Our thoughts lead us to have feelings which then lead to actions.

We always have a choice. We wouldn't get moving if we didn't think and feel like it, and we wouldn't eat well or sleep on time. Providing the right conditions isn't even half the job done. As we've mentioned earlier, for over seven decades, there has been talk of increasing physical activities. For way too long, we have been told that it needs to be done because it's good for us. When has that ever been the biggest motivator?

Also, when it comes to mental health, way too many of us are living in the past or are worried about the future. Our minds are overworking themselves, and we forget to live in the now. It's all about thinking.

3

Psychology

We think too much and feel too little.

—Charlie Chaplin[1]

We are definitely a lot more than a bag full of bones and some organs. We think. Thinking leads to feeling, which further leads to action. That's what makes us human.

As mentioned in the previous chapter, the brain is one of the three musketeers, and that's where the software called the mind resides, where thoughts originate. These thoughts define us and make us who we are. But as Charlie Chaplin pointed out, most of us have a tendency to think too much but not feel sufficiently. This lack of feeling leads to inaction. But then, there are those who feel excessively, leading to overreaction.

Although we may not admit it, most of us have been dealing with mental health issues to some extent. But they have surfaced in the pandemic and post-pandemic era, where our minds have been overworking but we simply haven't been able to translate those thoughts into appropriate action. We have been forced to spend so much time at home that we have all had the chance to think more. Even the best of us have not been spared. To be able to address our thoughts optimally, we need to first recognize and understand what we are thinking. There may be a problem or concern that we have, but probably, only when we recognize and understand our thoughts, will we have a chance of addressing them. The mind has a major role to play even in physical pain and diseases and, in some cases, can be the main cause. Yet, somehow, the majority of the medical fraternity have taken the mind for granted or have disregarded it completely and have only attempted to treat the physical component.

Words and language are extremely powerful, and yet, doctors and therapists tag people with exquisite diagnostic labels, without understanding the implications.

The problem with diagnostic labels is that people end up going to 'Dr Google' which throws back the worst-case scenario results for each of those conditions as that gets it to the top of the search list rather than the boring symptoms even though they happen to occur in most cases. Soon enough, without realizing, people start to experience what they've read about. We all get too engrossed in feeling sorry for our poor selves and run from pillar to post, looking for help.

As soon as you step back and, with a calm mind, look at the situation objectively, you'll start getting answers. You need to start listening to *your* story. You need to connect those dots and work on each of them. You have lived with yourself from the time you were born, and there is no one who knows you better than yourself. No, not even your current sweetheart or your parents. Then how could that doctor or therapist pass a judgement on your future after barely having a snapshot of

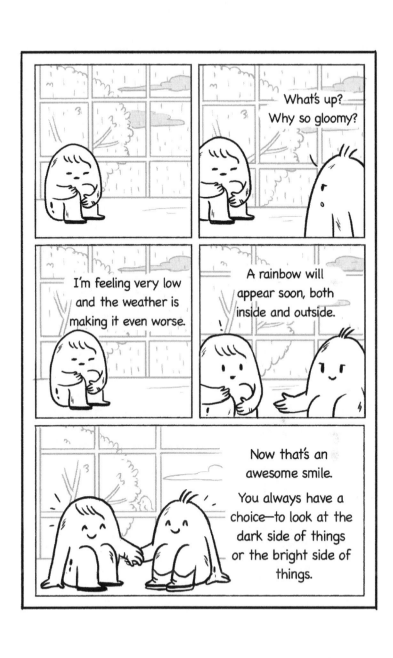

the situation they gathered from the 2–3-minute interaction with you? Think for yourself. Give yourself more credit. This means acknowledging the good times and the bad, the ups and downs, and everything in between.

We will not get into too many technical terms but will broadly look at what are the major issues that we end up facing. Our idea here is to enable and empower you, and not to confuse you further. As is the intention of the book, you need to take a proactive role in your well-being and not be dependent on anyone else. We have made a conscious effort to keep our messaging simple because psychology can get a bit too complex. But then again, as Charlie Chaplin said, 'Simplicity is not a simple thing.'[2] Or as manga artist Natsuki Takaya says, 'It's all very simple. But maybe, because it's so simple, it's also hard.'[3] For that, we have taken help from Purnima Sahai, a counselling psychologist.

Let's discuss things that hit us on a regular basis, things that we may not even notice. What we need to do is catch them early and address them when they aren't yet serious problems or haven't yet manifested into something else but are definite precursors to major issues.

Here are three things that one should definitely look out for:

Mood shift is one of them. All of us, at some time or the other, to varying degrees, go through our lows and highs. It's natural to have them but what matters is how high are the highs and how low are the lows, how often they come along, and if they come on with minor triggers, and how we respond to them and how they end up impacting our lives. It is also very important to recognize these highs and lows. Many of us do not even know when we are feeling low, or we deliberately avoid admitting that to ourselves. It is often our loved ones who can see these things before us, so do not take offence if someone asks whether you are feeling okay.

These mood shifts accompany physical changes in women a few days before and during periods every month and are known as premenstrual syndrome (PMS). Similar mood swings also happen during pregnancy and perimenopause. These are biological changes that happen because of alteration in certain hormones. It is perfectly normal to have mood shifts during these phases of life but too much of a swing can become problematic. This has, for too long, been a taboo subject that should now receive more attention so it can be dealt with better.

Mood shifts are by no means limited to women only. Weather conditions can have a similar effect. When the sky is overcast, we say that the weather is gloomy. It is because people feel low when it is dark and cold for long periods. When travelling to Scandinavian countries, there is an alarming increase in the mention of suicide helplines in in-flight magazines. Some areas there have no sun for a few weeks to months. Sunlight plays a major role in this change in feeling. This is the basis for a syndrome known as seasonal affective disorder, also known as 'SAD', where symptoms of depression can be more prominent in the dark winter months. The real-life equivalent of pathetic fallacy.

How we relate to ourselves and how we treat ourselves is yet another important behaviour to keep in mind. There are two common kinds: those who don't think very highly of themselves and outsource control; the other extreme who think a bit too much about themselves and assume that the world revolves around them. We need the right balance. We need to strive to think well of ourselves and be in control. We need to become our own best friends before we expect anyone else to become ours or before wanting to become anyone else's best friend. As a matter of fact, when you take care of yourself, only then are you capable of taking care of anyone else. So, it's not selfish to prioritize yourself and be in control of your life to whatever extent you can.

If we don't treat ourselves well, how do we expect anyone else to treat us well? It doesn't mean that we don't need support from others but we need to appreciate that they can never play the central role—that'll always be you. They can be there to guide you, but you have to be the one to act. Without your involvement, nothing changes, and definitely not for long.

Purnima Sahai shared[4] Ranjan Sethi's (*name changed*) journey. Ranjan, a professor of economics, has been a mentor for generations. He somehow found himself in a precarious situation. His name was proposed for the position of vice chancellor. Soon after, false allegations had been levelled against him by a colleague who was jealous of Ranjan's success. Ranjan, through no fault on his part, fell in his own eyes and started to avoid colleagues and turned down the position. This started affecting the quality of his classes as he simply couldn't focus on work. He had never been in a situation like this. He blamed himself for the other person making false accusations against him. After looking into the matter, the university gave Ranjan a clean chit, but he simply wasn't able to get back to his usual self.

Mahender Shah (*name changed*) had a different experience. One fine day, he had a bit too much to drink. He just wasn't in his senses. He arrived home past midnight. When no one responded to the bell, he yelled at the top of his voice asking for the door to be opened. He woke up the neighbours. When the doors were opened, he abused his wife and elderly father for the delay. He then told his wife to prepare dinner for him. She refused and walked away. Mahender slapped her. When his father tried to stop him, he too was slapped and pushed on the floor. Mahender threatened to kill both of them and broke the windows of the house. Luckily, neighbours intervened and told Mahender to leave the house.

Mahender's elderly father decided to side with his daughter-in-law and his young grandchildren. They were all scared for their lives. Mahender has been banned from coming into the residential society. Once sober, Mahender realized his mistake. He realized that this one act of his would lead to him losing all he loves.

When sober, he is a gentleman who speaks politely and respects his elders. But he has had a love–hate relationship with alcohol for over a decade now and has been struggling to give it up. He has been trying to make up with his family but his wife is clear that she wants a divorce and Mahender's father supports her. His father appreciates that Mahender has a serious alcohol addiction and needs to undergo de-addiction rehabilitation. But Mahender is now suicidal. He has fallen in his own eyes and simply lost the will to carry on if he loses everyone he loves. Of course, he messed up big time, but it is important that he faces what he has done and works on corrective measures rather than following an escape route.

On the last day of the wretched 2020 (i.e., 31 December) which had brought the world to a standstill, Rajat got this handwritten letter from Shashwati,[5] a patient of his from 12 years ago.

I am writing to inform you that I am doing great physically. My pain, which was all over my body, is almost gone. Yes, it does flare up once in a while but, it is not what it used to be. I am almost free of pain. I am also quite fit – bodywise and muscles stronger. Of course, I have had help with all of that but the reason I am sharing this is because I have never been this fit in my life and never as physically strong as I am now and I reached here after a rather rocky journey. I'm still on it but it started with you. Even though I first met you in 2010 and you gave me the advice then, I finally took it in 2015. I booked myself with a psychologist and my life has never been the same since. To put it mildly, my whole life, as I knew it, turned upside down and am still picking up pieces. I have lost a lot but have also gained some.

This isn't a sob letter. I guess what I am trying to say is that in the hell I have been through, still am (sort of), with all the loss, incomparable ones, I found a little peace, calm, breath and freedom from pain in all the PAIN.

I would have NEVER sought help had you not asked me to see a psychologist. I would have never gone myself because I never thought I was 'mad' and anyone else suggesting, I never would have paid heed. Infact, one doctor had asked me once 'if I was faking it all', after all my investigations came out normal but me still being on the bed and sick. I yelled at him. With all my love and respect for you, it still took me 5 years. Therapy changed my life – I don't know for better or for worse. Nothing on Earth would have ever prepared me for the shock I landed myself in. It was slow, painful death and bits of me are still dying. But, I am fit, strong and free of pain physically. I have also released oodles of body weight. It's like a magical transformation if you look from the outside.

I don't know for myself if all this was 'good' or 'bad' news. I am just sharing how it is. I came to you for my pain. So, I definitely want to share the great news that there is no more pain (well, almost none) and I feel great. But most importantly I want to say 'Thank You!'

You knew the pain wasn't in my body. It took me so many years to know. The delight of living without pain, I can't thank you enough.

Then there is threat perception (anxiety)—how we perceive fear or danger from a particular situation. A classic one is that we all know that we are going to die, but if we just get too worried about that and forget to live before we die, our lives would simply be miserable. By no means are we suggesting that you be careless. Every aspect of life comes with risks and we just need to learn to appreciate and recognize how to manage and live with this risk. An important one to remember during the times of the pandemic is 'say no to panic but say yes to precaution'. We need to balance the threat a situation poses and how we tackle it.

Today, too many of us live in fear of what has happened in the past and are too worried about what'll happen in the future, forgetting to live in the present. As they say, 'Do not let your past dictate your future.' After all, now is all we have.

We would like to share another person's journey narrated by Purnima. As the COVID pandemic began, Vidur Thakar (*name changed*) was one of those who went through a really rough patch. He had invested a lot of his own and his parents' life savings. He had also borrowed a huge sum from moneylenders as he saw the potential of his business growing big. But the pandemic had other ideas. His business went totally bust. Vidur lost all the money. He had to move back from Mumbai to his parental home in Delhi as he couldn't even afford rent for a one-room flat. Vidur's decisions had put the whole family in an extremely difficult situation. His father was upset and his creditors were giving him death threats, demanding that he return their money in a certain time.

Vidur had shared a broad outline of his story with Purnima over the phone before seeing her for the first time. Purnima was pleasantly surprised to see a composed, well-groomed, attentive young man, since she was expecting a tired, unshaved guy to show up. On being asked what his secret for staying sane under such tough conditions was, Vidur said that from senior schooldays, he had started to focus on his health. He would go to the gym, run, eat well, meditate and go to sleep on time. He had maintained this habit throughout college and when he started working. He had to maintain his routine to be able to perform at his peak at work. He didn't drop his guard on it even for a day. Even when everything fell apart, he stayed as calm as he possibly could and found a job. The salary didn't make a dent in the money he had lost but helped him with his routine and to focus on building back, one baby step at a time. Of course, Vidur needed help and that's why he sought help from Purnima. But he did a good job of holding himself together even in these tough conditions.

Then there are those who need to be guided to get back on track. Preeti Singh is one such story. An investment banker on Wall Street, she had to quit her job because of her back pain. She stumbled upon Rajat's book, *The Pain Handbook*, and then travelled all the way to India to be treated. She suffered from lower back pain in a foreign land and threat perception (anxiety) seemed to be pulling her into a downward spiral.

Common sense medicine helped her to get back up and help others too. Preeti explains:

It just takes one doctor to give you confidence and then you can work hard and get better. Being treated like a human with emotions and not just a physical body goes a long way and gives lasting results. And I was lucky to have found help!

As any young person in their late 20's, I led a very active lifestyle. However working on Wall Street as an investment banker, I spent long hours being glued to my seat. In 2014, I got severe lower back pain and was diagnosed with a herniated disc. After visiting a multitude of so-called "specialists", I wasn't getting better and had to go on disability and stopped working. Over that whole year, the pain discouraged me from moving and my muscles got very weak. I even developed sacroiliac joint pain. I was just 31 years old! And I could not sit for more than five minutes, could not stand for more than twenty minutes, and I needed help for many basic activities. Even after many months of physiotherapy sessions, I just did not find the relief I was looking for and felt very weak.

In 2015, I got pregnant and fortunately found a good therapist who helped me get strong enough to deliver the baby. Pregnancy and delivery went smoothly. However, after having the baby, I still had to rebuild my strength as I had not fully recovered from my original back issue. For many months, I took care of the baby lying down. I was not able to carry him either. I started developing neck stiffness and shoulder pain. The next few years were spent with frequent back pains and shoulder pains. I could not go out much, our social life reduced, and traveling for fun was almost close to nothing. It started affecting me mentally and I was losing confidence. I knew I needed more help. My son was my motivation and I had the drive to get better and get my life back to normal.

In 2020, my friend recommended that I see Dr. Chauhan in India. Before my flight to India, I read his book called "The Pain Handbook: A Non-Surgical Way to Manage Back, Neck and Knee Pain". It gave me so much hope and I immediately messaged him. He agreed to see me and I met him the day after I landed. He checked my muscles and the first thing he told me was, "You are ok. There is nothing wrong with you". All my MRI and x-ray reports were normal other than the herniated disc. He explained to me that years of muscle weakness and fear of movement had caused these issues and that I can get back to being fit again. He clarified a lot of my queries and recommended a plan.

I would like to mention that while in the US I did not have much help with the baby or housework. My husband was always there and very supportive, but with a small baby, it was hard to manage the day to day work while he was working. I used to be scared of doing new exercises as it would increase my pain and I feared how I would manage the home and the baby. I also felt low at times when I could not lift my son because of back weakness. All this caused a lot of stress and anxiety. I noticed that my neck muscles got tighter when I felt this way. Dr. Chauhan recommended that I see a pain psychologist first and then recommended a course of exercises with his physiotherapist.

I only had two sessions with my wonderful pain psychologist, Dr. Divya Parashar.[6] I explained to her what I had gone through over the past years and what was going on in my mind. She advised me that a lot of the pain comes from our minds and our emotions and that I should learn to let go. She taught me to notice how my mind felt when I got pain. I started *practicing her recommended advice for a few weeks and I tried not to worry or get stressed about pain. When slight pain would happen to the areas where I used to experience it in the past, I told my mind that it's ok and that I need to let go. I started realizing that the pain would actually eventually go away or the frequency and intensity of it would decrease. And that it was not as bad as my mind perceived it to be.*

I also started exercising under the guidance of Dr. Chauhan and his physiotherapist. I started going for walks and gained a lot of confidence. I even tried running, even though it was just a few meters. Being with my parents helped me a lot as I was mentally relaxed and knew my son was looked after. This allowed me to break the boundaries that I had created for myself and just focus on exercising. I realized that I could do more and more every day. Dr. Chauhan and the physiotherapist helped me with any questions I had and were there to guide me if I experienced pain. They assured me that when new muscles are being exercised, it is normal to experience some discomfort and the pain and stiffness would eventually decrease as I build strength. That was exactly what happened in the months to follow. The mental confidence that I got from them really helped me move to the next level.

It was definitely a journey of mind against my muscles. In the midst of coronavirus, I continued working with them online. The recovery was very slow in the beginning, but with their assurance I kept on working hard and took baby steps. Today I am much better and my back is much stronger. I am still building muscles and gaining strength every day. I still sometimes get pain but it doesn't scare me anymore. It took me more than five years but it did get better. I have come to realize that once we get past our mental barriers, physical barriers are easy to conquer. The pain does get better, muscles do get stronger and with a positive attitude and a drive to get better, you can overcome your physical pain. A little boost of morale from your doctor goes a long way. I really thank Dr. Chauhan and his team for helping me get my life back on track.[7]

After about six months, on Christmas in 2020, Preeti sent this message to Rajat from New York:

Thank you! Thanks to your help I'm finally able to fully enjoy myself with my family. This is the first year I had a normal life – simple things like bending, running, playing with my son, sitting and making tons of crafts, baking, which I am passionate about, putting diyas on Diwali to decorate for Xmas without pain and leading an everyday normal life! Baking is my passion and I can finally put that cake in the oven without help. And now that I can sit for more time, I can type! Finally started a blog for little kids to help them learn. https://www. facebook.com/therenewedmom/ All this equates to less time being in pain or laying in bed, less mental stress and getting life back on track and back to walking and exercising. And most importantly, I enjoyed that first snow, and could finally bend and make a snowman and snow angel with my son. Hurray! Thank you again![8]

4

Psychological Needs (The Human Givens)

For life to exist and survive in this world, water and air are crucial. Then comes the need for nutrition, which can be extremely different based on the species in question. All animals do build some version of a house too, although most other species do not go as far as we humans do. Once survival has been addressed, then the plan for any organism is to carry on the lineage, for which reproduction is crucial. Whatever needs we have, we need to figure out the resources to address them.

When it comes to psychology, what makes humans unique, as the name Human Givens (a holistic framework to understand how individuals and society function)[1] suggests, is that we are given solutions, rather resources, to address all our human psychological needs. We have mood shifts, low self-esteem, threat perception and other behavioural issues if our needs aren't met appropriately. It is only when these needs are met and balanced that we can have psychological stability and harmony.

The ideas below are based on our conversation with Dr Ivan Tyrrell, co-founder of the Human Givens Institute, who has done an enormous amount of work on psychology and human beings.[2]

None of this is groundbreaking for any of us. We are all very well aware of all of this, no matter what age, religion, education, etc. It is just that somehow, we simply forget to apply the same to our psychological needs.

There are nine emotional needs that the Human Givens model recognizes. All these needs that we have are a form of nutrition; too much or too little is bad for us. Besides quantity, we need to have the right quality too. No one need is any more or any less important than the other. Effectively, there is no hierarchy. Also, all these needs overlap each other and are interconnected.

Sense of Autonomy and Control

Pretty much from the time we are born, and probably even before that, all of us want to have autonomy, which is a sense of control over ourselves. We want to have that sense of independence and freedom to make our own decisions starting from which toys we want to play with, to clothes, food, cars, house, religious practices, profession, life partner, etc. However, there are times when we must rely on others to make decisions for us, for example, when we are babies. But we must grow to develop independence and autonomy.

We like to be in charge, even though we know that there is only so much control we can have. It could be a football or a cricket match, running, relationships, exam results, salary, or one's career path. You simply can't control how the weather will be or how others will behave with you. Examiners, referees and bosses can behave independent of your efforts. We need to hope for the best and be prepared for the worst. All we can and should focus on is doing our best. It is important to remember that you should only be concerned with that which you can fully control and influence the outcome of. If we put all of our efforts into this approach, rather than worrying about what we cannot control, we would probably not feel as stressed and anxious.

On the other hand, there will be those who lack the need to have control. They would think that no matter what they do, nothing would improve, so why bother. But then again, if you don't take the shots, you are guaranteed to miss them all.

None of us want to live a life which is out of control, but a balance must be found. For some, this balance can be found early in life, but for others, it can take a while. Experiences as well as relationships help us to reflect on control in its many forms and how we can adjust our approach for the future.

Some would want to be in too much control of themselves, everything that happens to them and everyone around them. A classic example would be a running coach. Of course, they create running plans with the best of intentions which some runners would follow and others might not. That's because there are all kinds of people out there. Some would follow and yet not get to the desired results because of injuries or even weather conditions. We don't want running coaches who are control freaks telling everyone to change everything else in their lives and start living like them. If you don't know enough about who you are coaching, about their lives and their past, then it is difficult to work with them. Coaches are not you and you are not them. At best, they can guide you and help you to make decisions and take actions that best suit you. Then, it's up to you. After a point, you can't even control injuries as they are inevitable in running as they are in life. All your plans and exercise can do are reduce those injuries. The important learning for life is how people bounce back from those injuries when the supposedly unexpected happens rather than thinking that life would always happen exactly as planned. And yet again, that's why running is so like life.

Safety and Security

The need for safety and security too comes into play from the time we are born to our very last breath. Probably, we feel the most secure when we are a foetus in our mother's womb. After that, we all want to have a safe environment to live and grow in. If that environment doesn't feel safe to us, we let our rational human brain be overpowered by the insecure mind, and start feeling anxious, fearful and stressed.

If you are obsessed with security, you wouldn't want to take a risk. You wouldn't want to start a relationship or start a new business or even cross the road, because of the fear of something going wrong. You might as well put on a helmet and a life jacket while you spend your lifetime staying at home. You'll not want your loved ones to venture out either or take even the slightest of risks. This behaviour is not healthy either for you or those close to you.

Human beings have only achieved what they have by taking risks. Again, it is a question of balance. Even at night, when you go to bed, there is no guarantee that the floor wouldn't collapse or the roof won't fall on your head. But it is a reasonable assumption that they wouldn't. We need to become comfortable with taking risks but not taking extreme risks ranging from financial, to physical to emotional, among others. It is through life experiences that we develop a sense of when and how to take risks. It is just that we all have a different 'barometer' around taking risks. Have a think for a moment . . . do you need to adjust your 'risk barometer'? It could be one way or another, but it is important to reflect on this regularly through life.

You might join a running club or become part of a tribe for the sense of security, a need that might have been missing from your life even without you realizing. There is nothing wrong with it. You will soon be offering the same security and comfort to someone else picking up running or exercise.

But if you are totally obsessed with that security, you'll not want to push yourself and take a few risks. That'll stop you from trying anything new, like running longer or pushing yourself harder and faster. Or maybe, the fear of not wanting to raise your heart rate too much because your family member, friend or even your doctor may have told you that it's not safe to have your heart rate above a certain number. This concern also comes through stories that you would have read in the newspaper about something happening to someone else, like death. Most people with such a concern end up staying at home and not getting started. They are dead long before their expiry date.

There will also be those who lack this sense of security and push themselves too hard, especially without appropriate training. Injuries amongst runners is a good example. Build a solid base and gradually get to where you want to be. An extreme example would be running a race like La Ultra—The High, without any practice or training just because that sense of security is missing. You want to just land up in Ladakh and run the next morning. This could help you graduate a little sooner than it was otherwise planned by the almighty, if there is one.

Status

No matter what our designation or role may be in an organization or in the family, we all like to be valued and respected by others. This applies to all, and all throughout life. With loss of status comes loss of self-respect, a sense of inadequacy and a feeling of worthlessness. It can become difficult to get out of this low self-esteem and to recognize how you can be valued again.

Whereas excess need for status, no matter what or who you are, leads to a pathological megalomania. Such people are a dime a dozen in today's world, and simply think a bit too much about themselves, ruining all relationships, whether it be at work or home. These are often people who have a high sense of autonomy but rely on making use of other people for their own gain. Becoming delusional about one's status is harmful first to your own well-being and then to everyone else impacted by you.

It helps to be humble and appreciate our insignificance, but at the same time, recognize that we are the most important to ourselves first and then to those who truly love us. So be kinder to yourself and those around you. Once we recognize that and come to terms with it, we will be at peace with ourselves and be able to lead a more meaningful life. As we have said previously, only when you look after yourself can you begin to help others.

You might be in an important, high-flying position now, but it gives you no right to behave like a total crackpot to those on their journey up. Don't forget where you started from. Be humble towards others before expecting the same for yourself. Sadly so, enough of them are found throughout life.

There are also people who let others run them over even though they have themselves accomplished a decent amount, just because they have low self-esteem. That is not okay either. If you don't respect yourself, no matter what position you have at work or in personal life, why should you expect any different from others?

Running is a good example of how status can be used in a good and bad way. When our advice is valued by fellow runners, new and old, it gives us runners an identity. We are accepted and respected in running circles. As runners, we use social media platforms like Facebook and Instagram to reach out to the world out there to share our advice and to expand our status. In the running community, not many care about your professional and personal life or standing. After all, when you are running with a group of people around a park or on the road, you are all running in the same direction and towards the same destination. We are respected for our running exploits, so we start giving it priority over everything else. Running gives us an identity, which for some of us, was lacking earlier, a need that is important to all of us. But yet again, too much or too little is the problem.

After having run a few races or maybe after having accomplished 'good times', some become delusional. Unfortunately, some people get 'above their stations' very quickly and think they are better than they are. Of course, they have improved and are now good at running, but that doesn't mean that they need to treat others with disgust or as low lives while throwing around their weight about how special they are.

If you forget where you started from and are not humble towards others who are on their journey or probably just starting, it gives you no right to behave like a total wally. Sadly so, like in life, enough of them are found in the running community too. If you are one of these people, learn to be humble and respect your journey so that you can respect others. If you are a person who has been 'run over' by one of these types of people, try and stand up to them and remind them that they are runners just like you.

Privacy

We all need our privacy to reflect on our thoughts and ideas. Sports, especially repetitive endurance activities like walking, running, cycling, swimming, etc., can help you with that me time. After all, we are creative, reflective creatures.

When we do these simple repetitive activities, we tend to go into a trance where parts of our brains will consolidate our experiences even when we are not thinking about them.

Lack of need for privacy doesn't let us reflect on our thoughts as we need a quiet environment with ourselves to do that. It'll lead to us being anxious and stressed with unresolved issues in our heads. On the other hand, if we need too much privacy, we will simply push people away. Being social beings, it'll backfire, leaving us alone, and soon enough, lead to loneliness too. A few could do well by being hermits, but most would struggle being cut off completely from other human beings. It's only through interaction with other human beings that most of us learn and evolve.

Running has often been called 'meditation in motion' because that's 'me time'. After all, we are reflective creatures. Even if you are running in a group, the excitement of being in a community you like and that likes you back, shuts off all the other noise from the professional and personal fronts that bother you, letting you unwind. Also, even if you are running in a group, more so when you run long, you tend to get lost in your own thoughts. It helps you think. This degree of privacy while running gets you into a running trance, helping you consolidate other experiences even when you consciously don't think about them.

But yet again, some like being solo runners. Personally, we are of the opinion that if you enjoy your company, get on with it. But it is very tricky to last very long on your own as we are social animals and, so, we need the right balance.

If you have no desire for privacy, you tend to miss out on the me time, and the benefits of running such as unwinding and reflecting start to dwindle. At times you can't figure out why you haven't started to like running as much as before. That is why we emphasize the need to know why one picked up running and why one runs.

Although running is a great example of privacy as a form of meditation, it may not be for everyone. The important thing is to recognize what level and form of privacy works for you. This might be a 'traditional' form of meditation in a quiet and dark room, or it could be climbing to the top of a mountain. We must pay more attention to this need and take the necessary time to dedicate ourselves to the mode of privacy that works for us. This leads us to the next need.

Rajat is someone who has been an introvert and loves his own company. Running has been a perfect companion for him. He has a relationship with running that most struggle to understand till they discover running. His running doesn't judge him, no matter how fast or slow, long or short. It's just there. And that's exactly what works for him. When he is out running, not thinking about anything, that's when he gets his ideas. The trick about running is to not even think about running when you run. Just be. Let go. That helps you get into the Zen zone, in sync with your surroundings. After all, running isn't about running itself, it's about life. Once you are comfortable to let go while running, it translates to a sense of comfort of not being attached with anything in life too. It's always a journey of self-discovery, with no destination.

Attention

We all need to give and receive attention. As a newborn baby, if we don't get attention, we could starve and die. On the other hand, to raise children, we need to give quality attention for good upbringing. Again, too much and too little attention leads to lifelong issues, messing us up big time.

There are some people who are attention-seekers and all they want from you is attention. It is very unpleasant to be on the receiving end of that. They are just too needy. It could just mean that they didn't get enough attention when they were young. It's now spilled over into their adult life and they just need attention from people all the time. This can be excessively draining. It could very well be the exact opposite—they may have been given excessive attention and now expect it throughout their lives.

The same applies to those who seek little or no attention whatsoever. They are comfortable in their own company.

On the flip side, they don't end up socializing enough and struggle to make friends (too much privacy). This is why we talk about striking a balance so that needs are in harmony and one is not pushing out another.

In our personal opinion, both of us being introverts (we think so anyway!), there is nothing wrong with that if you are comfortable, but it does make it a bit difficult to survive in this social world. As Robert De Niro's character in the film *Heat* says, 'I'm alone, I'm not lonely.'[3] It is important to recognize that, and if need be, work on changing from lonely to alone. Since most people are not hermits enough to be comfortable with being alone, there is a need to work on social skills. The trick is not to try too hard, focus on looking for like-minded people. They are always around.

Runners, like all human beings, have a need to give and receive attention. That's one reason that motivates runners to join different running groups and socialize with running mates even outside of running. They get attention and give attention. Attention that possibly had been missing in their lives, both personally and professionally. Think of the attention that runners get in a park from the other people that are walking by, or even a mass marathon, where there might be hundreds or thousands of spectators motivating everyone to keep going.

Posting selfies and photos of other runners on social media serves this need. We all do things to fulfil this need. Some of us may also exaggerate our exploits on social media, making the audience think that we are better than we are. We are of the opinion that society has now become sick of what social media influencers have achieved and can't stop talking about. It doesn't interest the world any more. Even if you have had a podium finish or done some amazing times, after a point, besides yourself, it doesn't matter much to others. Becoming too needy for attention ends up pushing away folks who were possibly motivated and inspired by you. But then again, running just for social acclaim is a problem too. Running more than you have trained for, just to get attention, and also pushing others to do more than they are ready for, soon leads to disaster. Injuries, both temporary and permanent, come visiting. The same applies to running faster as well. You need to repeatedly revisit the question as to why you got started with running? If the fun and joy is missing, you are totally off track, figuratively and literally.

When you are a needy runner in a running group or in a race, you end up messing up everything for everyone else around you. Everyone starts to ignore you. At times, just one excessively needy person is enough to mess up the experience for everyone else.

Race organizers and club administrators give attention, due to the nature of their roles. They, besides everything else, may find themselves (or put themselves) in these positions to fulfil their own need to gain attention, and that drives them to do even more. This is not a criticism, but rather an honest view of these positions of 'authority'. It is not only in races but happens in all forms and levels of organizations.

Emotional Connection

We all have a need for an emotional connection with at least one person. Some of us need a lot more than one. We expect them to be biased in our favour. This could come from parents, siblings, grandparents, spouse, partners, children or friends.

You first need to be your own best friend before expecting others to be your best friend. But generally, lack of need for intimacy in life could leave you lonely, where you have no one at all to share your secrets with and unload your concerns on. The comfort that there is someone unconditionally out there for you is missing and that could be daunting. However, it is a lot easier to work with than it sounds, and we believe it is worth working on.

Excessive need for intimacy and dependency on any individual is a problem too. All who we have ever known or will know, will die. When our loved ones die and if we are excessively dependent on them, we suffer for far longer than we should. The same applies to all relationships. They, too, come with an expiry date. We all respond differently and it's okay. It is through life that we experience different emotional connections and learn how to connect and disconnect from these emotions.

One big reason for people picking up running is for the emotional connection. You meet people with similar interests and make lifelong friends and even love at times. In this virtually connected world, it is a need that is totally missed for most. It is very difficult to share and feel emotions through our 'smart' devices. Emotions come with a feeling, but pixels on a screen somehow fail to pass it on and do not allow for intimacy that is often needed.

Again, it is very important to not miss out on the bigger picture.

It could also be that you are so obsessed with your running that you end up ignoring your loved ones who have always stood by your side through thick and thin. We could also be ignoring issues that exist throughout the world, something like COVID-19. During the COVID-19 pandemic, it has been observed way too often that running friends gather together, of course because they love each other's company, with no regard for distance or masks. Soon enough, all of them get infected, spreading coronavirus to families and friends as well.

We need to appreciate the fact that we are a very important unit of society. Ignorance, denial or being oblivious to things happening all around us can have a detrimental effect on people we love. It's good to have emotional connections and to care about other people in this selfish world, but let's not be blindsided to the bigger picture.

Community

We are all social beings and have a need to be part of a bigger community. We all desire to have a sense of belonging where the community embraces us without being judgemental. This could range from political thinking and religious thinking, as well as fans of sports teams and sports communities where you do activities like running and cycling as a group. These could be other social and cultural groups too like reading, debating, dramatics, etc. We all want to belong to a tribe, a cult. It gives us an identity that we are probably not getting and being appreciated for by the rest of the world. This makes us value our community even more. After all, why do you think all these types of groups and societies exist? It is because we have recognized a need for them. Through our associations with them, we eventually end up having friends from the same community. Even before COVID came along, virtual communities were already picking up, but they have become the norm today. As we have discussed, these communities can have benefits but could also fail to recognize important aspects related to our needs.

Those who lack a need to belong to a community are considered reclusive and are not able to relate to others.

An excessive need to belong to a community too ends up making one a blind follower of whichever community one belongs to, without questioning anything. This is rampant today and has been the case even before. When the term 'brainwashed' is used, we are talking about such individuals who have lost their own sense of identity and capability of thinking logically for themselves. Suicide bombers belong to this category. When we put such communities ahead of our own and our loved ones' well-being, it is detrimental to us as individuals and to society. When things go wrong, which they have a habit of, it's only your loved ones who'll stay by you, so please don't push them away.

Being part of a wider community, in this case a running community, is yet another need. We want to belong to a tribe. Running makes us belong to a local, regional, national and even global running community, both real and virtual, courtesy social media. Anyone across the world who is a runner shares the same feeling and all runners can recognize that. But we shouldn't become too obsessed, addicted and dependent on the running community.

Some experience that in the early days of joining a running club. They tend to start ignoring their immediate family because they are too focused on their running mates. This ends up creating friction in marriages and families. Some like being solo runners, and we are of the opinion that if you enjoy your own company, get on with it. But it is very tricky to last very long on your own as we are social animals. So, we need to have the right balance.

Achievement and Competence

We all have a need for a sense of achievement, as to what we have accomplished, and a sense of competence, as in how good we are at what we do. This gives us confidence in our abilities and adds to our self-worth.

People who lack a sense of competence or achievement end up having low self-esteem. They feel very inadequate about themselves no matter what they accomplish. This could be triggered by parents, siblings, teachers, peers, co-workers and partners never being happy about what one does. We need to realize that our challenge is always against ourselves and the objective is to be better than that. As long as we give it our best, we are doing well. This is where it is important to set goals, but goals that are achievable and set for us and not for other people. Some have this feeling of not being good at anything and just being average. We are all good at something, something we like, and we need to discover what that is. It's not about others. We need to become comfortable with ourselves.

On the other hand, people who think they have achieved too much and consider themselves extraordinarily good, tend to have egocentric traits, not necessarily a healthy state to be in. They are found in all walks of life. What they fail to understand is that there is always someone who is a lot better than them. As a matter of fact, when you look around, there will be a lot of people better than them. So, it helps to be humble. We can always learn more, which is a fascinating property of the human brain. The idea of 'student for life' is one that most of us do not really subscribe to. Once we finish our education and training, we think that we know everything we need to know. Recognizing that we can always learn more will help us to achieve a lot more.

Running marathons is a phenomenon that has caught on only in the last decade or so in India. People who weren't running earlier tend to forget why they picked up running now, i.e., for the joy, and soon focus solely on speed. Most don't miss a chance to show the world how good they are. In 2021, Sania Sorokin, a Lithuanian runner, broke the 24-hour record, covering 309.4 km, averaging 4 minutes 39 seconds per km. Most who brag about their speed and don't fail to put others down can't even maintain that pace for 30 minutes. And that's fine. But bragging and making others feel bad is not. We should all simply strive to be better than our previous selves. Healthy competition is important but we should be mindful to not let it take an ugly turn. A lot of different running events have emerged in recent years with the sole purpose of bringing back the fun element to it. For example, trail runs, challenge runs and obstacle runs. These events often have different aspects beyond basic running including resilience and bravery. They have been designed well to align with many of the needs that are outlined in this chapter.

There is another aspect to think about. If you desire to win an Olympic gold medal in 100 metres but can't run that distance in faster than 11 seconds, you will keep fooling yourself. Lots of lives are wasted because more than children, it's the parents who want to have trophy children to talk about at their kitty parties or boardroom meetings, even when children aren't enjoying the sport. Most children enjoy it when they pick up a sport but tend to lose interest when it becomes excessively competitive. We need to go back and look at that.

A runner's desire to be good at running might not fit with what they are capable of achieving. There would be well-intentioned people who would argue that we are being discouraging here, but in life, we need to be able to distinguish between reality and optimism. Some of us, no matter how hard we try, end up taking an awfully long time to run short distances. But we keep persisting because of our need to compete. The realization of what we can achieve is important. We need to figure out what we are good at. There is nothing wrong with running short distances in a long time, but we must be aware of our limits and capabilities.

Mass running events are amazing because, unlike any other sport, prizes are not limited only for the winner or the top three. All participants who get to the finish line get a finisher's medal, certificate and even T-shirts at times. Most of the runners get all excited about these medals and certificates. The new ones definitely do. It's a massive motivator for them to carry on and strive for more. Some races put time or completion limits on their events and decide whether to award prizes on this basis: ultimately, this is at the organizers' discretion, but everyone should be awarded for their own respective achievements.

Prizes give a sense of accomplishment, and of competence. Runners are then likely to post selfies and photos of other runners on social media, announcing their accomplishments to the world. That sense of competence—that they are good at running—is a need that needs fulfilling. We have the desire to be the best, better than all the rest, at everything we do, including running. We all do. But our desire to be as good might not fit in with our ability, no matter how much training is put in. Some friends who know Rajat well might point out that he would never tell someone that they are not capable of something.

Rajat admits that he can't dance to save his life. Darren is also very nervous about dancing at parties and weddings unless he has lost some of his inhibition by drinking some alcoholic beverages. There is no doubt that by shedding our inhibitions and with practice, we'll become better. Soon, though, we'll plateau off. But when it comes to running, things are different. For Rajat, once he gets into a rhythm, he can float. He can just talk to the wind and it has nothing to do with how fast he is going. It is slightly different for Darren, who finds it more challenging to run longer distances. For him, he feels free and in rhythm when he is running (relatively) fast over distances less than 400 metres!

There can also be a disconnect between what we enjoy doing and what we are good at. Prateek Gupta, who joined the Run & Bee running mentoring programme,[4] acknowledged the fact that he could possibly run fast 20 years ago, but now, even though a lot slower, he is enjoying it a lot more.

Just as Tom Cruise's character in the opening scene of the film *Top Gun* is reminded not to sign cheques that his body can't cash,[5] the same applies here. There could be injuries that could have happened even though you did all things right or maybe because of overtraining. Or it could be that you simply can't run any longer or faster. When people go through what some refer to as a 'midlife crisis', they often pick up things like running. This is when things can go wrong—when you think you are still fifteen years old and nothing can stop you. You have a choice. You could either feel sorry for yourself, blame everyone who cares about you, and not do anything besides grumbling and messing up good, long-term relationships. Or, you could get back up and slowly start working on the basics, one baby step at a time.

A lot of factors come into play for the results to be a certain way. Some are in your control and others are not. We need to strive to become our best, putting in our best efforts. A few setbacks shouldn't upset us. Rather, they prepare us even better for the world out there. Becoming better than our old selves isn't only about numbers. It's about the effort you are putting in, which means that we must learn to recognize that different outcomes can relate to success and achievement.

It is like the game theory which suggests that your best efforts are responsible for the best outcome. Nothing else is anyway in your control. Just that those outcomes might not match what you desire. We need to appreciate that when we run, our main objective should be to become better than our yester self, not against all others in our running group and in every race we participate. This is the philosophy of the Dalai Lama who said, 'The goal is not to be better than the other man, but your previous self.' Some of us, if all things were perfect and in sync, can possibly run 10 km in under 35 minutes, but others might make it in only 45, 60 or even 90 minutes. So be it. You can't beat yourself to death over it. But you definitely need to put in your best effort. And become your best, doing justice to yourself.

As for the races, runners who don't make it to the finish line need to be recognized for their efforts. The effort put in during training as well as in the race itself needs to be recognized. In running, the most dreaded term is 'DNF'

(Did Not Finish), a term that brands you as a failure if you don't get to the finish line. Some treat it as a failure for life, messing up their lives beyond running, and letting it affect their professional and personal lives. As Kieron Berry, a La Ultra participant who carries on running even after having undergone heart bypass surgeries on three different occasions reminded us, DNF should stand for 'Did Not Fail'. And that, we think, is very powerful. Let's recognize effort a lot more.

Meaning and Purpose

As Mahatma Gandhi said, 'Whatever you do will be insignificant, but it is very important that you do it.' This seemingly simple quote puts it all together really well.

To continue in this world you need a reason to carry on, otherwise, it is all worthless. Human beings are probably the only animals who know that life is temporary and that eventually they are going to die. Possibly, we are the only animals who have the awareness of being aware, and that's probably why we need a reason and a purpose, to carry on in life. It's okay to have our own purpose which could mean nothing at all to the other person. There are three aspects to this.

Firstly, we have a need of being needed by others, be it raising a family or being an integral part of a work or sports team; as a teacher in school or as a nurse or doctor in a hospital; or helping a community in some way, etc. It gives us a meaning and reason to carry on in life.

Secondly, learning new mental or physical skills helps us to look forward to the journey of life. When we get to a certain stage in life and have been doing some activities for a while, we either reach a point where we can't improve any more—it's not challenging enough or has just become boring now. Then, we need new challenges for things and life to be meaningful. As much there is the talk of 'midlife crisis' as we have said before, it has nothing to do with a particular age. It's about what stage of life you find yourself in. These activities could involve starting to learn chess, starting to run, getting to the gym to become stronger, travelling, learning a new language, crafts, dance or music too. When we think about it, it is not at all about the activity, but about rediscovering ourselves through giving ourselves a new lease of life, literally.

When in 1986, nine-year-old chess prodigy Josh Waitzkin won the US National Primary Championship, everyone thought he was going to be the next Bobby Fischer. At the age of eleven, in a simultaneous exhibition, he drew a game with chess grand master Garry Kasparov. For the next decade, Waitzkin dominated the scholastic chess world. But, because of several reasons, chess stopped giving him the kicks it gave him earlier. From a cerebral game like chess, he switched to the martial art, t'ai chi ch'uan, that challenged him. Here too, he excelled and ultimately earned the title of world champion.

In his book *The Art of Learning*, Waitzkin admits, 'I've come to realize that what I am best at is not Tai Chi, and it is not chess. What I am best at is the art of learning.' This is something that Darren always tells his students, 'If there is one thing that you learn when studying at university, it is "how to learn".'[6] If you figure out the best way that you learn things, you can literally apply yourself to anything. This is especially the case in the age of the Internet when there are free tutorials and enough information online to help learn absolutely anything.

This holds true for all of us, even if it's not aimed at becoming a world champion. When professionals from across fields pick up running in their twenties or after, in spite of not being physically active before, and then carry on with it, it is because running challenges them and they can then appreciate their progress over time. The beauty about running is that it's always you v/s you.

Thirdly, it is often quoted that being connected with some sort of political, philosophical, religious, national or spiritual ideas that appear to you to be bigger than your own self, inspires someone to do more than they think they are capable of doing.

One of the main reasons for most people choosing to run is to fulfil the need for finding meaning in this life. Human beings, for as long as we know, have strived to find the meaning of all the suffering that comes along in life. If we are going to die anyway, then what is it all about? We all need a higher meaning to get on with life.

Eons ago, Buddha left the comfort of his royal life in search of the same. If you come to think of it, he walked—a lot—long before Forrest Gump[7] came along, and definitely before Aamir Khan ran across India as Laal Singh Chaddha.[8]

When running gives us that purpose, that meaning, suffering becomes a lot more tolerable. We push ourselves to the goals we set ourselves in running. This works in one of the following three or more ways.

- **By Being Needed:** When we have a sense that we are needed by other runners, whether as running mates, running groups or for organizing running events, it serves our need of being needed by others. It is reason enough to get up every morning and get on with life. Even if it's 10 per cent of your entire personal and professional life at any given time, it helps you stay upbeat. It more than compensates for feeling low with other parts of life.

Again, getting too involved in running, and prioritizing runners and running over family and friends that have been there for us through thick and thin, may feel like the right thing to do in the short run but by the time realization hits home, it could get too late.

But then again, running-related friendships can last real long. It's a bond that can cut across cultures. Rajat knows runners from twenty-four countries who have participated in La Ultra. They all highly respect each other for what they have gone through together in those extremely tough conditions in the high-altitude desert of Ladakh. But they don't put these relationships over everything else. Most of them will always be there for each other but they also prioritize their personal lives above all that. It's that fine balance, yet again, that is important.

- **By Learning New Mental or Physical Skills**: When you start running totally afresh or after having taken a decades-long break, it fulfils the need to learn or relearn both mental and physical skills as running caters to both. As a child or youngster, we just ran without thinking much about it or because we loved it, but when we are older, reintroducing ourselves to running helps us bring meaning to life.

We could be doing well in professional life but it may no longer be exciting or it might be falling apart and running helps to give us direction through a new sense of excitement. It could also be that we have gotten sick of the rat race at work and sitting in those cubicles. Having those me times helps us connect better with ourselves.

Rajat has, time and again, witnessed the joy very successful people get when they pick up running from scratch, almost like children. It's because, subconsciously, they are using these new experiences in running as metaphors for life. Here, they have an opportunity to set things right.

- **By Being Connected in Some Way with Political, Religious, Sports Groups or Spiritual Ideas that Are Bigger than Ourselves**: To some runners, over a period of time, running connects at a higher level, bigger than the self. Running has a cult feel to it. There will always be some running mate whose wavelength will sync with yours. In today's social media world, you'll form a group with like-minded people. Through your running group, you satisfy the need to discuss other things that make sense to you.

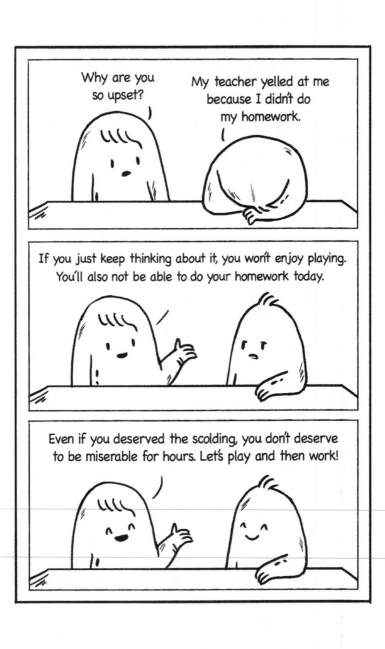

5

Psy-Phy: The Psychology of Movement

By living happy, and also having one and a half hour a day exercise programme, I haven't been sick in fifty years. Want to be well? Be happy and have an exercise programme.

—Patch Adams[1]

Too many of the good folks in the 'exercise-fitness-sports' and 'mental health' space, somehow, don't value the other one enough, so we can't really blame doctors and therapists who don't value exercise and mental health enough. But both of them go hand in hand. They have to. After all, the brain, the hardware for the mind, resides in the human body. No matter what, it simply can't be independent of the body. We need to look at them together and what the psychology of getting someone to physically move is.

Understanding Exercise Psychology

Prof. Ekkekakis points out that exercise psychology is not a new field.[2] It is more than five decades old but our doctors and other allied health colleagues don't know of its existence. They talk about psychology in pain and exercise as if they've discovered something new. To take it one notch up, even most psychologists aren't aware of it. It is unfortunate that the sports-exercise medicine and science fraternity are not asking some fundamental questions, like the ones given here, and, instead, carry on making assumptions.

Does exercise really make people feel better?

We all know (or do we) that exercise is good for us, and still, we don't do it. Why?

Exercise has been found to be the most effective and safest of treatments for psychological issues like depression and anxiety. Still, not enough of it is prescribed or done for these conditions. Why?

Babies and children love playing, running and jumping around all over the place. When they start going to school, somehow, everyone is keen on them following a structured programme without appreciating that we are all unique and different things work for all of us. Almost all children love to be active, but not necessarily all of what is being done at school, and almost definitely not the way it's being done. Giving it structure and making it compulsory makes sure, even if done for now, that it is not carried on for life. Soon, the same fun activities get boring or even seem like punishment. Sometimes, they actually are punishment. The philosophy of Montessori education tries to align with what young humans should be exposed to by promoting self-directed activity that supports physical and interactive (with others) play. Unfortunately, most early years education settings (nurseries, kindergartens, etc.) become too rigid and push children into routines that they are not ready for.

In school, you could have possibly picked up sports because of the love of it, but as you get better, the primary thing that everyone wants to focus on is you becoming better, and why not. We all should do justice to what skills we have. Here is when the coach or physical education teacher comes in, who, even with the best of intentions, is starting to make everything more regimental with the intent to keep you improving. The fun is slowly going out. As you start moving up from the class team to the school team and then further up to represent your district, the pressure is on performance, not on fun and enjoyment. By now it's become a chore, if it wasn't already one.

Elders, parents and coaches are often yelling at you or each other so that your results can improve, whether justified or not. They all want you to win because they had a dream to win that for themselves, their school, district, state or country. You don't really matter. Darren can recall playing football (soccer) for a local team when he was a teenager, where every week he would witness pushy and often angry parents either shouting at their children, other's children, or each other! This was all in the pursuit of what they thought would help their children perform better. The ones who excel at a sport because they are talented or enjoy doing it are the only ones who carry on doing it. They are the fortunate few. They have mentors and coaches who help them enjoy the journey rather than get bothered by the results.

This is about elites who move up the ladder quickly. Most systems, even in most good schools focusing on physical activities and sports, are structured in a manner that the above average, average and below average who don't make the cut for teams, end up becoming the audience. Not being appreciated for your efforts and playing only because it's part of the system soon just becomes a chore too, more like punishment. It is a known fact that many girls stop taking part in any form of physical activity when they leave school. There are, of course, many reasons for this, but one reason is that they are not allowed to take part in sports and activities that they enjoy and feel comfortable about taking part in on their own.

Rajat gives a lot of credit to what he has become to a boarding school he studied in—Wynberg-Allen School in Mussoorie. His elder son too went there and now his younger one is still studying there. Running is an integral part of this school, with morning runs being a crucial part of the daily routine. In 2016, Rajat started a half-marathon for the school with shorter categories of 5 km and 10 km. At the end of the annual events, Amisha Sachdev, a senior student, walked up to Rajat and thanked him. 'Today is the first time that I have got a medal in anything—a finisher's medal. Otherwise, it's always limited to the top three. I have tried to be sporty and worked hard to get into teams to be recognized but I am just not good enough. Thank you for appreciating my effort and everyone else who ran today, whether they came first or last.'

And this is a school that would easily be in the top 1 per cent in India that focuses on holistic development of children by integrating sports really well.

The problem is not only about recognition and encouragement of being active for all but using these same activities not for encouragement but for punishment. That complicates matters even more.

As recently as 2014, the UK Department for Education's publication, 'Behaviour and Discipline in Schools—Advice for Healthcare and School Staff',[3] had the following recommendation under Behaviour and Sanctions:

'When poor behaviour is identified, sanctions should be implemented consistently and fairly in line with the behaviour policy. Good schools will have a range of disciplinary measures clearly communicated to school staff, pupils and parents. These can include:

Extra physical activity such as running around a playing field.'

This advisory is thankfully now missing from the UK's Department of Education but the teachers remain the same. It's ingrained in them to use physical activities as punishment because the same was done to them. And when it comes to India, it's far worse. But of course, it's a system handed over to us by the British.

Whether you were punished like this in school or not, once you have a negative connotation associated with physical activity such as running, squats, skipping, etc., that's what it'll be for life. A punishment.

We did a survey on social media (Twitter) and found that 86 per cent of adults now remember having been given physical exercises like running or being made to do squats, headstands or handstands, touching their toes, ragra-patti[4] or made to stand in poses like a murga, putting their hands up, kneeling on the floor, etc., as a punishment, whether it was at school or home. 27.5 per cent were given these punishments 10–100 times during their schooling and 16 per cent were given these punishments over 100 times, or at least that's what they recall.[5]

Doctors can be as good as they are in prescribing exercises, but when adults try to pick up physical activity later on in life, whether it is to address a chronic disease like diabetes or to get back to being healthy, it's not out of pleasure, but as a punishment for being a bad person. It is similar to a binge of yummy but sugary stuff being followed by a 'punishment' of an evening walk. There is almost always a negative connotation associated with exercise and movement, and that needs to change. That can't help sustain physical activity for long. In any case, when anything is prescribed, we think of awful tasting medicines. Do we ever think, 'Wow, time again for yummy meds!' We have to make exercise and movement fun, else it will not last long.

* * *

You would think that maybe people don't like to exercise because of the negative connotation associated with it. But it should be common knowledge that being active and sporty is good for health, and we would all be super active if we had sporting facilities around. After all, there are at least a couple of news items pretty much every day about some research demonstrating this beyond doubt. But is it? And if it is, why isn't everyone running, cycling, swimming, working out at the gym, skating, playing football, hockey, cricket, bungee jumping off cliffs, etc.?

According to a recent US study,[6] 54.7 per cent of people strongly agreed that it is important to engage in regular physical activity. Of course, there were an additional 30.3 per cent who somewhat agreed to the same. This does mean however, that there are people (15 per cent) who do not recognize the importance of physical activity. Only 40 per cent strongly agreed that a walkable neighbourhood, i.e., one

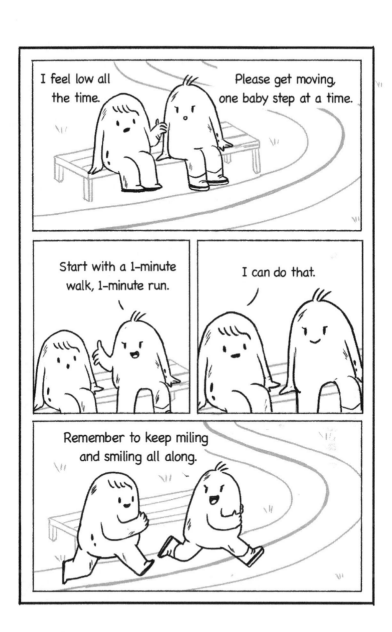

that is safe and easy for people to walk to get somewhere or one that is safe and easy to walk for fun, relaxation or exercise is important. And only 31 per cent agreed that both regular physical activity and walkable neighbourhood are important.

So, not being aware that physical inactivity is a health risk factor, but not even appreciating that walkable neighbourhoods are important for health is a major problem. It baffles us. We simply can't get our heads around this, but we need to think deeper and in a collaborative fashion. It translates to less than 10 per cent people around the world being active to meet the physical activity guidelines that have been globally agreed upon, i.e., 150 minutes in a week. Although these numbers might be brandished around by the World Health Organization (WHO), they are not even enough.

A 2007 report by YouGov and the British Heart Foundation[7] found that 62 per cent people would not do more exercise even if their lives depended on it. How can any amount of information and knowledge then help that? A third of them were active enough to do the minimum recommended exercise but only 4 per cent found exercising fun. How can it then be sustained for life?

Remember the proverb 'You can lead a horse to water but you can't make it drink'? Can we simply leave it there or is it something that passionate advocates of physical activity, exercise and sports are totally getting wrong and if yes, why?

Prof. Ekkekakis raised a fundamental question.

'How do you sell something where all you can promise is a small benefit? Nobody has managed to market something desirable by promising that it would be tiny. Unless it's a bitter pill. Essentially the message you are communicating when you say that you only need to do this tiny bit, not too much, is that this tastes terrible but you'll only need to do [a] tiny bit of it, so just close your eyes and just tolerate it, you can then get on with the rest of your life that is pleasant. We are effectively saying that exercise is unpleasant, boring, tedious, monotonous, painful, unpleasant.'[8]

That is exactly what everyone is trying to do. 'You only need to do 30 minutes of exercise only 5 days a week. Even walking qualifies for it.'[9] It almost sounds like an awful-tasting pill that you need to take because it is good for you.

But sadly, that is the message being given by the WHO, followed by all well-meaning associations, organizations, institutions and bodies looking to make us as active and fit as we possibly can be. Our messaging has been totally wrong. We are all excited and passionate about spreading the benefits of exercise and movement without knowing a thing about the psychology behind it.

Prof. Ekkekakis has an interesting question: Would McDonald's be able to sell any burgers if they had a similar pitch?[10] They always talk about how yummy and big the burger is, and with it, you might even get an unlimited amount of cola. They are selling pleasure, not displeasure, but in the exercise fraternity, we have been busy selling displeasure. And we think it'll do the magic because we are throwing all kinds of data every day at homo sapiens of all kinds.

In Rajat's boarding school, exercise and running were also punishments. It's not surprising then that most of his batchmates didn't carry on being physically active even though they are all from a school in which sports was an integral part of education. They all had a negative connotation attached to exercise and running. It wasn't something you did because you loved it. As luck would have it, Rajat loved running alone more than talking to his peers or playing with them. He would get excited when, as punishment, he had to go around the field a few times. Somehow, most institutions even today can't make the connection.

In 2003, at a Higher Education conference organized by the British Medical Association, Rajat had inquired about sports and exercise psychology as a field, but the staff member drew a blank. We guess that's because of two things. Firstly, even today, doctors are not recognizing the role of psychology enough. Secondly, all experts, even today, are working passionately in their own fields, but in silos, not making enough of a connection between physical health and psychology. We should have recognized, with exercise being so ingrained in our natural survival, that psychology would be very closely linked to how we are motivated to do it. Although this seems simple, we have made it vastly complex.

As much as McDonald's burgers aren't the best for you, there is something very important to be learnt. The famous McDonald's catch phrase, 'I'm Lovin' It', is probably one of the greatest marketing feats in history. When they ran the TV adverts, they would use a catchy musical tone prior to an audible, 'I'm Lovin' It'. They ran this advert for just long enough so that everyone would either be saying it in their head when they heard the tone, or they would even be saying it out loud. Now comes the stroke of genius, as they then removed the audible, 'I'm Lovin' It', so that everyone would just say it of their own accord.

We have to get fun, pleasure and simplicity into healthcare, physical activity, exercise and sports. Ask anyone who smokes, drinks alcohol and consumes drugs as to why they do it even though they know all about the side effects. It's because it makes them feel good at that moment. After all, we belong to a society that enjoys instant gratification.

As Dr Adams recognized so early on, we need to move to be happy, and joy in movement helps us keep moving for life. This combination is needed to keep us in top physical and mental health, and even when things do go off for a bit, the combo of happiness and movement gets us back on track sooner than it otherwise would.

Dr McGonigal was helped immensely as she was a student of group aerobic exercises years before she was a student of psychology.[11] This gives her a totally different perspective compared to psychologists who don't understand the body enough or exercise trainers who don't appreciate the mind enough. In her book, she talks about how ultra-endurance athletes, when fully exhausted, focus on putting one foot in front of the other, rather than think about the finish line which could be a long way away. These athletes could be running 11 km, 22 km, 33 km, 55 km, 111 km, 222 km, 333 km or 555 km at La Ultra in the inhospitable conditions of Ladakh in the Indian Himalayas or participating in the Ironman triathlon anywhere around the world, but it is the same story. This confidence and courage comes from both the brain and also from irisin, an 'exercise hormone' that is manufactured in our muscles when we are physically active to an optimal level. It gets released into the bloodstream and goes on to stimulate the brain's reward system, making it reach a state of tranquillity. Some would call it the 'Zen zone'. You don't have to be doing ultra-distances to experience the benefits. These physical activities can be walking, brisk walking, jogging, running, swimming, cycling, strength training, higher intensity strength training, etc. The idea is to do more than what you are used to. It could be about higher intensity, duration, a better form, longer distance, etc. You should be mindful of not suddenly increasing any of this but gradually building it up.

Irisin and its family of hormones have a neurological role as they protect the health of brain cells; help the brain generate new neurons, decrease the inflammation in the brain, and play a role in reducing a number of neurological diseases, including Parkinson's.

Irisin is also known to have natural antidepressant and anti-anxiety features, which is probably why Rajat sees these benefits when he suggests his patients start moving and, gradually, start pushing a bit more every week or two. Irisin is also known to have a role in metabolism, burning fat as fuel and regulating blood sugar. When muscles contract at an optimal level, these hormones, on being released, are a motivation booster. For that very reason, they were labelled as 'hope molecules' in the first scientific paper that was written on them. Like a drug, our body does get used to the amount of this hormone that is circulating following exercise, which is why we need to challenge ourselves, not only to do more, but to do different forms of activity. Our muscles will respond differently and, therefore, the timing and amount of such hormones will also change. This could mean trying different forms of running like sprints, longer distances, etc., or trying resistance training.

The Magic Called 'Discipline'

In September 2018, Commander Abhilash Tomy from the Indian Navy had made it to the front page of almost all national newspapers.[12] He was participating solo for the second time in the Golden Globe Race, where he was supposed to circumnavigate the globe in a non-motorized sailboat. Soon, he found himself caught in extremely rough weather; his boat was damaged and he was thrown off the mast.

He was unable to move his legs and his back was very stiff. The satellite phone was in a bag which he was not able to reach. He had a satellite texting device, which he used for sending messages to the race organizers, suspecting a back injury.

He was stranded in the middle of nowhere, with Perth, Australia, being 3500 km away and the closest island about 200 km away but with no means of rescue. It was two days later that the Indian Navy was able to contact him and only on the third day was he rescued by a ship.

He was advised spinal fusion at five levels because of multiple fractures in his spine. The big concern with spinal injuries is loss of function and sensation in body parts supplied by nerves at the injured level and below. In his case, it would be about below mid-torso. If surgery wasn't done, there was a high chance that he would not walk again.

As an adventurous person, as much as you want to live, you are always thinking about getting back to doing what you love. He was unsure about the surgery but reluctantly went ahead with it 2 weeks later. In such cases, surgeons advise a conservative approach where exercises can be delayed and there is extensive bed rest. Long days in bed can lead to major muscle wasting that delays recovery by months.

The game changer for Abhilash was that he got moving 3 days later. He wasn't straining his injured area but moved unaffected body parts like toes, thighs and neck and arms.

Care needed to be taken not to overdo exercises as the injury could become worse.

Over time, he started doing more resistance exercises and picked up on hydrotherapy in the pool. In two and a half months, he was moving around comfortably and his strength was back to almost 80 per cent of where he was before the injury. Besides the surgery, the fact that he decided to start moving quite early helped immensely in his recovery. It's yet again very important that it's done gradually.

Either extreme inactivity or overactivity are both recipes for disaster, not only in extreme cases like this but even with non-traumatic back and knee injuries that most runners face.

The important takeaway is that there is no magic exercise. Magic lies in the discipline of moving and gradually pushing harder. Effectively, a good exercise is one that is done, that too with discipline, not one that looks very good and complicated, but is not done.

Small Steps

Prof. Ekkekakis has a couple of similar observations, 'An important message, in my opinion, is showing what gain will be there in a set period with those minor gains doing minor activities daily.'[13]

'Effective exercise is only the one that can be sustained over the long haul. Limited period of time to accomplish goal x, and the exercise will be so extreme and difficult that I can't incorporate it in regular life, you soon stop it and all the adaptations reverse pretty soon. When participants from *The Biggest Loser* were assessed after 6 years, they got back to square one after having initially lost all that weight. You can push people to the max and cause spectacular adaptations quickly, if they don't injure themselves, or don't die. Unbelievable spectacular changes will happen, but those shouldn't be of interest to us. Our goal should be long-term changes, lifelong behaviour changes.'[14]

In a different context, when Rajat started with La Ultra, it was 222-km-long. That's extremely long for most to comprehend. The majority of Indian runners were excited about it but couldn't ever fathom running that distance. Once the distance was reduced to 111 km, Indians started to take part. They not only finished 222 km and 333 km in 2019 during the tenth edition of La Ultra, but three Indian runners stood at the start line of 555 km, and one managed to finish it as well. That only happened because the step's height was reduced, else it seemed too far away to ever reach.

In 2019, another distance, which saw a lot of resistance from purists in the La Ultra core team, was introduced. The distance of 55 km was considered unworthy of the name. But what that did was get a lot more people to participate and now they could dream of doing 111 km in Ladakh. After a 2-year lull courtesy the pandemic, in 2022, the plan is to make those steps even smaller and introduce 11 km, 22 km and 33 km distances so that every runner can dream of participating in the race.

To Get the Best of Your Exercise, Be at Peace with Yourself

Thirty-five-year-old Nisha (*name changed*) sat across from Rajat in his consultation room and coyly admitted that for over a decade, she had tried all kinds of programmes but had failed over and over again. But then, something happened.

She didn't get very far with all the things she tried. Her exercises ranged from group classes, personal trainers in all kinds of gyms, running, following online programmes, having personal coaches and even being part of multiple running groups, and doing yoga of all kinds, vipassana; from being unorganized to organized ones over weeks, diets from low carb–low fat to low carb–high fat, to paleo, vegan, Atkins and intermittent fasting.

She was committed to getting better but failed again and again. Her blood tests were normal. In her professional life, she was doing extraordinarily well. Her times for running half-marathons were far better than most men. Her children were doing well in school. Her husband shared responsibilities, like teaching their children, and doing all household chores.

But she was tired all the time. She wasn't happy even though she was popular on social media for her image in all fields she got involved in. She was broken, both emotionally and physically. She was unhappy. What was going wrong?

A chance visit to Leh during the off season made her come face to face with herself. She happened to spend a few nights out, looking at the Milky Way. Initially, she loved the beauty but soon, it started making a lot more sense to her. It suddenly sank in that she was insignificant.

Suddenly, her materialistic achievements, which others respected her for, which she literally ran after, meant nothing. It was this sense of insignificance and impermanence that she felt happy about. She had been resisting way too much. She realized that she needed to let go. Like our own planet just floats in the cosmos without having any false impressions about oneself.

As soon as Nisha started to do things for the fun and love of it, it all started to make sense to her. It was no longer for anyone else or what they thought about her.

She connected with her deeper self. She realized that she was fighting too hard. She decided to let go and just be. Similar to 'kintsugi', the Japanese art of repairing broken pottery with lacquer dusted with powdered gold, rather than running away from her problems, she started to treat her aches and pains as her own identity and build up on those blocks rather than throw them away.

Now, Nisha and her family take time out for physically active family vacations where it isn't about going to some posh exotic locations, but where they spend time with themselves, getting to know each other and going for treks and long walks together. They have often gone on long drives together, without the rush of getting from one location to another. Without being preachy, Nisha has spread her learnings to her loved ones. Now they mile and smile together as a family.

Even in the cosmos, or as the basic rule of physics goes, matter can't be created or destroyed. All life forms on our planet exist because of heavenly bodies. When we start using the lessons of life as lessons themselves, only then will we improve. Else, it's all a waste of time.

6

Sleepin' It Off

Laugh and the world laughs with you; snore and you sleep alone.

—Anthony Burgess

Forty-five-year-old Rajeev Lingaraju (*name changed*), a senior executive at one of the top Forbes 100 companies, was an extremely active person. A good runner, he used to run for over an hour a day and spend an equal amount of time every day in the gym, pumping iron like no one's business. On weekends, he would play either golf or lawn tennis. He always took care of what he ate. He would get timely annual medical check-ups and was in top shape. Rajeev's family doctor would always praise him for his fitness.

In any boardroom meeting, he was extremely sharp and would pick the fine print apart. He was great at reading the body language of his peers and using it to his advantage. His work required a lot of air travel. He was happily married to a woman who was equally accomplished in her professional life. They had two children just about to finish school and

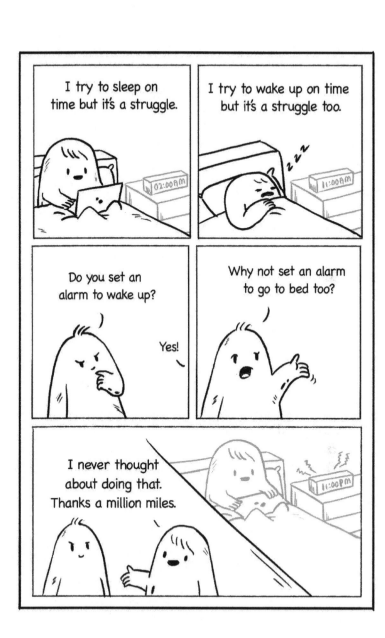

were doing very well overall. The couple always found time to help their children with schoolwork. He always told his wife that no amount of pressure stressed him out and that he would soon become a senior executive in his company. He had the right work-life balance. His colleagues, folks in his friend circle and extended family envied his overall success.

One fine day, he collapsed while he was running 5 km at a relatively easy pace. A passing police car noticed him falling to the ground. He was rushed to the best hospital in the city, which was less than 10 minutes away. Sadly, he was pronounced dead on arrival.

What could have possibly gone wrong? He was in the top shape of his life and that was for all to see. He exercised and ate well and wouldn't let anything get to him. What more could he have done? Sometimes, we need to look beyond the obvious.

We sleep for approximately one-third of our lifetime. 'That one-third of our sleep time actually controls two-thirds of our wakeful time, so that's very important, because our wakefulness, both in terms of the physical and mental health, is not going to be very sound if that one-third of our lifetime is not suitable to and conducive to solid restorative sleep,' says Dr Deepak Srivastava, professor of medicine, sleep, pulmonary and critical care, University of California, Davis School of Medicine.[1]

Even though Rajeev exercised a lot and ate well, he just didn't sleep enough. After all, there are only so many hours in a day, and he was just too busy to sleep. He would sleep for a maximum of 5 hours, with 4 hours being his average. He was always telling everyone that sleep was for losers and that he'd sleep when he was dead. Even when he did sleep, it was erratic. He did not have any fixed sleeping time. Very often, he had late nights either because of work or parties, late dinners even when at home, red-eye flights two to three times a week, etc. His autopsy revealed that he died of myocardial infarction, also known as heart attack.

Such stories are becoming more and more common in today's world. Being aware of that, and when a series of such episodes happened in relatively younger employees, one of the 'Big Four' accounting firms in the world approached us to put together an awareness session. Apart from us covering the physical and psychological aspects, one of the top cardiologists was on the panel as well. He was a likeable chap who, unlike most cardiologists and doctors in general today, wasn't heavily focusing on pharmaceutical and surgical approaches. He gave a lot of importance to nutrition and eating habits. He was interested in healthy lifestyle habits, and it wasn't just a fancy word for him to drop in passing.

Yet, when it came to the role of mental health or physical fitness, he somehow didn't think there was much of a role for experts in the field. Sleep was nowhere spoken about. And that is the problem we have observed across the board amongst the good guys in medicine. Somehow, they don't think about all the four verticals that interest us, i.e., move, sleep, mind and food. Making the connection between these four is a distant desire. And that's where it becomes very important for you, the reader, whether a non-medic, sportsperson, medical student or a practising doctor, to make yourself more aware.

So, what was it that Rajeev could have done better? To begin with, he should have been simply sleeping longer. We should target to sleep for 7–9 hours a night. A lot of us would argue that 4 hours or even less is enough for us and we don't need any more sleep. But if you haven't suffered the consequences of lack of sleep, you have no clue what you are missing out on. All your life, you've been functioning pretty well with 4–5 hours of sleep, but come to think of it, you probably could have achieved a lot more in life, especially peace of mind, had you just slept a bit longer every night. Just give it a shot. Try it for a month or two, and if you think it is not adding anything to your life, go back to your old self. But do try it for a month or two. No less.

Lack of sleep over long periods is known to reduce cardiovascular performance by 11 per cent. If someone has accumulated 30–36 hours of sleep debt, it is enough to cause a significant detrimental effect on cardiovascular performance. For example, if instead of 7–9 hours, one sleeps 2 hours less every night, over 15 days there would be a deficit of 30 hours. Think of it like hanging on a cliff side, holding on to a rope for dear life. The edge of the cliff keeps cutting the rope but you don't realize the situation you are in till the last string of the rope snaps and you tumble down the gorge. That's how sleep debt works. It's all good until it's not any more. Just like you, out of the blue, your physical or mental performance goes tumbling down. Imagine that for just not having slept well and adequately. As it is, inactive, sedentary people don't have great cardiovascular fitness, and if the heart's performance is reduced further, it can pile up soon to cause disaster. We have to remember that sleep is the time when our body has a chance not only to rest, but to recover and regenerate. As we sleep, our body has an amazing way of releasing certain hormones which allow the body to repair itself. It therefore makes sense that if we do not sleep enough, we are not allowing our body enough time to repair.

For those like Rajeev, who are extremely active physically and under a lot of work pressure, the heart is already working at maximum capacity. It needs all the help possible. When sleep deprivation leads to further load on the heart, the potential consequences should be no surprise. Such incidents have been increasing at a remarkable rate over the last two decades. And when the inevitable happens, i.e., death, it makes it to the newspapers or at least to the morning WhatsApp messages. The sedentary and sloppy people in the family and friend circle will suggest how exercising kills people and how all of us have a certain quota of breaths, so why waste them on running, cycling, swimming, working out at the gym and doing other exercises and sports.

As common as it is, what doesn't make it to the newspaper or social media is when a sedentary person sitting on the sofa, checking Instagram and Facebook every minute, while binge watching films on the smartphone, tablet or television and munching on potato chips and pizza with extra cheese and gulping down family-size aerated drinks, suddenly collapses and dies of a heart attack.

The message is simple. Exercising is very important, but your nutrition, mental health, rest and recovery, and sleep are equally important to have optimal benefits. Ignoring any one of them spoils the delicate equilibrium. Yes, we all have a certain quota of breaths but none of us have any clue how much that is. By leading an overall healthy lifestyle, you can maximize your chances of getting to that number while leading a high-quality life.

Let's go back and understand first as to what Dr Srivastava was alluding to when he said that 'one-third of our sleep time actually controls two-thirds of our wakeful time, so that's very important, because our wakefulness, both in terms of the physical and mental health, is not going to be very sound if that one-third of our lifetime is not suitable to and conducive to solid restorative sleep'.[2]

Yes, it's being repetitive but it's worth pausing and spending time to let the above statement sink in. Whatever physical activities you do, whatever you eat and whatever you think (or at least you think you think) happens during that wakeful stage. If your quality or quantity of sleep hasn't been optimal, it affects both your physical and psychological health and performance. But which one is it that it affects first?

We posed this question on LinkedIn and Twitter. Over 150 people responded. More than half got it wrong. Before affecting you physically, lack of good-quality sleep first affects you psychologically. And you don't even realize it because physically, you are still on the top of your game. Your mental functioning decreases twice as fast as your physical functioning. Because you can carry on physically performing optimally for longer, most of us think that our decision-making is good too.

Even though more and more people now, either intuitively or because of reading articles, know of the importance of rest and sleep, sleep is still the first one to be sacrificed, as was the case with Rajeev, without appreciating how serious the consequences could be. Whether it is students in schools and colleges, entrepreneurs, corporate employees, housewives, elderly or elite athletes, society takes pride in compromising on sleep or pushing others not to sleep. In hospitals, junior doctors are expected to do 24 to 36 hours. Wrong decisions can directly be fatal for patients being attended to. Students in all kinds of institutions are already stressed because of competition and the workload. They sleep less to address the stress and anxiety. Rather than helping the situation, lack of sleep makes the situation worse. Not only do they perform worse as compared to if they had slept well, but they end up having suicidal tendencies. This situation is rampant in top institutions around the world.

Until I'm six feet under
Baby, I don't need a bed
Gonna live while I'm alive
I'll sleep when I'm dead
'Til they roll me over
And lay my bones to rest
Gonna live while I'm alive
I'll sleep when I'm dead

While growing up, one of Rajat's all-time favourite songs was Bon Jovi's 'I'll Sleep When I'm Dead'.[3] Even though he would run for 2 hours a day, trying to better his time each day, he wouldn't sleep enough. After all, sleep was for the weak. On top of that, in pop culture, it was popular that Albert Einstein only slept for 2–4 hours, when he actually slept for 10 hours a day. But then, there were others like Nikola Tesla, who has been known to sleep only for 2 hours every night. These are exceptions, rather than the norm.

Rajat picked up ultra-running in 2002 when he was in London and realized for the first time that on days when he slept for 8 to 9 hours, he was able to perform better in running, even if it meant running 4–5 hours. On days when he slept for under 6 hours and then ran even an hour, apart from not being able to run as fast as would have liked to and yet exerting himself more than he normally would, he felt tired throughout the day. His advice since then has been that sleep is as important as training itself because it's during recovery that your body and mind adapt and make the most of the training you have done.

To see the impact of deprivation of sleep, a study[4] on recreational endurance runners found that after 30 hours without sleep, their endurance performance reduced. What makes it interesting is that these runners thought that the effort they were putting in was the same as before, if not more, assuming they were going as fast as before, when they had actually slowed down. With our own race in Ladakh, we've noticed that runners running over days for 222 km, 333 km or 555 km did better when they rested well, as compared to those who didn't rest as much and thought they were working harder. Their intensity of work seemed to be harder than what it actually was. When you sleep, your mind rests as well, recovering for the next day, and when you restart, whether running an ultramarathon, playing a sport, writing an exam or going to the office, you are calm and can make better decisions.

Coming to non-elite athletes, a survey done by Philips[5] found that 72 per cent of Indians do not get enough sleep. In India, overweight people are often called 'healthy' and those who snore while sleeping are assumed to be in deep and sound sleep. Going by that assumption, Kumbhakarna, younger brother of Ravana, would be the epitome of health and fitness in Indian culture. As we all know, that is just not the case. Kumbhakarna was tricked into asking for 'nindrasan' (bed of sleep) even though he had planned to ask for 'Indrasan' (seat of Indra), so he could become king of gods. In Ramayana, when the battle was going on between Rama and Ravana,

Kumbhakarna was snoring away to glory till he was abruptly woken up from his deep slumber. He sleepwalked to the battlefield, creating havoc for a tiny bit but soon after that, it was game over for him.

It's then interesting to note that snoring can be an indication of an individual suffering from sleep apnea, a sleep disorder where breathing pauses for several seconds, at times, even minutes, multiple times a night. That stops you from having a good quality of sleep and wakes you up sooner than your body needs, at times, gasping for air. When you wake up, you aren't rested enough, definitely not fresh enough to take on the next day. It is estimated that one out of every five (19 per cent) Indian adults experiences sleep apnea. Most people do not even know they are suffering from this condition. In fact, it is often their partner or other family members who notice that the loved one has stopped breathing. If someone does get this recognized as a long-term condition, in severe cases, they can be prescribed a continuous positive airway pressure (CPAP) device. The device effectively keeps the airway open so that when the person is sleeping, they are still able to breathe.

Whether you are suffering from sleep apnea or not, if your quality and quantity of sleep is not optimal, it affects you in ways that most people can't even appreciate. It is no surprise that people with sleep apnea have daytime drowsiness and chronic fatigue (for years), which is double compared to those who have had a good night's sleep.[6] Sleepiness and tiredness throughout the day leads to difficulty in concentration impacting productivity at work and home. Half of those with sleep apnea see an impact on their personal relationships.

If you think logically, when your body and mind are not rested enough for long periods of time, it definitely has an impact on your overall health too. People with poor quality and quantity of sleep are at a higher risk of heart disease, high blood pressure, diabetes, obesity, low testosterone levels, stroke, neurological diseases, chronic pains in the neck, back, knees and even in the whole body. Overall immunity is low in someone who hasn't slept enough, increasing their chances of getting infections, more worrisome in this COVID era. There has also been a recent study,[7] which suggests that heart health is better with a bedtime between 10 p.m. and 11 p.m. Yet, it is not often that doctors or therapists ask or talk about sleep, leave alone listen to your detailed sleep story and make the necessary connections.

Seventy-year-old Priyanka Narang (*name changed*) was booked for lower back surgery for chronic lower back pain that had been interfering with her quality of life for over 2 years. Just a week before the surgery, her husband wasn't home. She ended up sleeping for over 9 hours. Lo and behold, when she woke up, there was minimal to no back pain. Narang couldn't figure what was going on. How was she suddenly better?

The surgeon had not bothered to ask her what her day was like, how long she slept and about the quality of her sleep. Even though she is wealthy and can afford all kinds of luxuries, she still washes all the clothes by hand and not in a washing machine. The couple don't have help to cook food; Priya stands for long hours doing all the kitchen chores. This is because her seventy-five-year-old husband feels that his clothes don't get cleaned properly in the washing machine and no one else makes food better than his wife!

To add to that, Priya ends up sleeping for just 4–5 hours because she likes watching soap operas after her husband goes to sleep. But in the morning, she has to get up before her husband to get him his bed coffee. No one realized that all she needed was some rest and a good night's sleep. She cancelled her surgery and has been relatively pain-free for over a year now.

Before going any further, we first need to understand the history of sleep. Humans supposedly used to sleep for around 12 hours a day in two chunks of six hours.[8] All this changed with the commercialization of the light bulb in 1880 by Thomas Edison, who had patented it the year before. Like a successful entrepreneur, Edison didn't only give the light bulb to the world but figured a way to make a shitload of money by developing an electric meter to track the consumption of electricity by each consumer. So, the next time your electricity bill gives you a heart attack, you know who is to be blamed. As for the light bulb, Edison had merely taken English chemist Humphrey Davy's idea (1802) and improved on it, remarkably.

Before the light bulb was available to the masses, sleep in humans was regulated by natural light. Our ancestors slept when the sun went down and it was dark and were up when the sun came out and it was bright. There was a schedule for sleeping and waking time that changed naturally through the year. Temperature and seasonal change contributed to the sleep cycle. Even today, after all the artificial interventions, our body functions, including sleep-wake cycle and levels of alertness to mood and digestion, have biological variations or rhythms over the 24-hour cycle called the circadian rhythm. 'Circadian' is a term derived from the Latin phrase 'circa diem', meaning 'about a day'.

These variations or rhythms throughout the day are natural waves of internal processes which regulate and respond to the sleep-wake cycle. Such processes are predictable and get repeated based on our behaviour and the interaction with the environment within a given 24-hour period. Such rhythms can be affected by exposure to sunlight and artificial light from all kinds of gadgets, our physical activities and exercise, our stress levels, and activity patterns, as well as eating behaviour.

Our circadian rhythm is inextricably linked to the rising and the setting of the sun. In reality, in modern society, this means our exposure to sunlight, i.e., when we go out in the sun. Within the brain, there is a 'biological clock' which receives messages from the eyes when detecting light. This part of the brain helps to regulate the hormone, melatonin, the 'sleep hormone'. When exposed to sunlight in the morning, the amount of melatonin decreases, and therefore, we receive a signal to wake up. In the evening, when it becomes darker, melatonin increases and we begin to feel sleepy. With extensive exposure to artificial light, our sleep-wake cycle goes out of whack.

We don't even need to go that far back. In India, even a few decades ago, most cities too didn't have electricity supply 24/7 and our circadian rhythm was doing just fine. If you haven't experienced it, your parents or grandparents would have told you stories about how they slept early and got up early. Without thinking much, they were just following nature. It was artificial light that changed sleeping patterns. As soon as there was availability of artificial light throughout the day, our days became longer. We were now starting to sleep for about 8 hours in one single phase rather than twice or thrice in 24 hours, as pointed out by Prof. A. Roger Ekirch, professor of history at Virginia Tech in the United States and pioneer in researching pre-industrial sleeping patterns.[9] Poor melatonin, the sleep hormone, already had no clue as to how to go about its work. And that was till a couple of decades ago. Now it's even worse.

A few years before the turn of the century arrived satellite televisions and smartphones that wreaked havoc on our lifestyle. Even before the introduction of the satellite television in every household, prime time television programmes used to be aired at 9 p.m. and most people, at the earliest, would only go to sleep at 10 p.m. Today, pretty much everyone has a smartphone that has apps which are a television and more. It is now pretty standard that people go to sleep the next day, i.e., past midnight. In India and all countries north of the equator, 21 June has the longest day and the shortest night. It's also called as the summer solstice. In 2021, the sunset on 21 June was at 7.22 p.m. Imagine the sunset at 7.22 p.m. on the longest day by when we should have had our dinner and got ready for sleep. In the winters, on the shortest day of the year, i.e., 22 December, at an average, the sun sets 2 hours earlier. But most of us only go to sleep after 10 p.m.

Today, phones have definitely got smart, but they have made us pretty dumb. Our sleep has gone for a toss. We are eating pathetic food at odd hours. Even if it's good, healthy food, it ends up being too late and close to sleep. We are moving a lot less than ever before. And society's mental health is at its worst. This cocktail is a recipe for disaster. We need to make these connections because no one else is going to do it for us.

Before the light bulb changed everything, our ancestors would listen a lot more to their own body. They would rest and sleep even during the day when needed, not bothering too much about deadlines, unless, obviously, they were the ones on the deadline, i.e., when they were the hunted rather than the hunters.

Some cultures still have a legacy of afternoon naps, such as Spain or our very own Goa. The short nap after the midday meal is called 'siesta'. Local shopkeepers there wouldn't care too much about what kind of business they could lose, but if it is siesta time, it is time for them to pull their shutters down. After all, if you can't rest when you want to, then what's the point of running after money! Aren't we all working our backsides off so we can eventually have peace of mind?

Many among us take pride in working a certain number of hours in a day, or of not having slept for long hours. But how does it help if your productivity is going down the drain during all that time? If and when you feel tired, you need to listen to your body and rest. And when you get up after a short nap of 30 minutes, at maximum 45 minutes, you are as sharp as you can be, concentrating fully on the task at hand.

Rupinder Chopra (*name changed*), an active seventy-nine-year-old woman suffering from back and knee pain, consulted Rajat. She improved a lot after getting on to a supervised exercise programme under a seasoned musculoskeletal physiotherapist. She admitted that she didn't have to take a single pain medicine over the past month. She only complained of tiredness and fatigue very early on in the day, and then felt that way throughout the day. On prodding deeper, she shared what had happened the day before. She was sitting on the sofa and having her coffee. The next thing she knew, she was flat on the couch and had spilled her coffee. She coyly admitted that she had passed out. She was distraught and embarrassed. She had been the one who was always in control of things, not only in her life but everyone else's around her too. An older adult having a sudden onset of fatigue sensation could be worrying. One would immediately think the worst. It didn't make enough sense. In a previous consultation a month before, none of this was reported. Back then, pain was her bigger concern. Was this a new thing?

The most exciting thing is that if you listen to the patients, they almost always have the answers. You need to just let them speak. They want to tell you the solutions. All of us find it challenging to share our problems with ones who are close to us. We all prefer to open up in front of strangers because they won't judge us. Or, at least, that's what most assume. If only we had someone who could hear us out.

> Rajat: Please tell me what's bothering you? What's going on
> in life? I have all the time in the world. Please take your time.

Such a simple statement can sometimes engage the patient more than ever before because it shows concern. It shows that you are interested in them and not just in their pain. It definitely doesn't happen in a 5-minute consultation, which has become a norm the world over. But rarely do you find such doctors today.

Rupinder felt a lot more comfortable.

> Rupinder: You know, I'm sleepy all the time. My fear
> is that I will go to sleep while I am driving. It's just that
> because of the lockdown I haven't been driving at all.

At least there was a shift in the conversation from being tired and fatigued to being sleepy all the time. That acceptance helped. It didn't seem like an intrusion into her personal life now.

Rajat: Please tell me more. Tell me about your sleeping habits and routine.

Rupinder: I go to sleep by around 10 p.m. and get up by 6.30 a.m. I do get up once around 2.30–3.00 a.m. to use the washroom. Most of the time, though, I don't end up sleeping after going to the loo. Even if I do, it is only for an hour at max. You see, I have to be up and about at 6.30 a.m. and get on with my routine. I then feel sleepy throughout the day, starting from 9 a.m. itself. I know that even a 10–15-minute nap can make me feel better, but I avoid it. If I go off my routine even by a slight bit, I get very anxious as I think the sky will fall and crash over my head. So, I don't end up lying down even for those 15 minutes during day time. I'm just staring at the ceiling from 3 a.m. onwards, waiting for 6.30 a.m.

Rajat: Ah. Thank you for that, ma'am. That helps immensely. What I will say next is not going to be comfortable, but I must say it. I know that you like to be in control. All of us do. Pride is an important characteristic that we value. But ma'am, what if you go to the toilet and a similar episode happens? Next thing you know, you are on the floor. That fall could lead to a hip fracture, something totally unwanted. Even though now we can efficiently deal with such things and get you back to being active, it could also take us a while to get you up and about. Even worse would be you hitting your head against the washbasin or the floor. And as your fear of driving goes, that can even be fatal. I apologize for being so dramatic about this, but it is essential for you to understand how a simple solution can prevent these unnecessary incidents from happening.

Rupinder: Thank you so much. I needed this. There was no nicer way to do this. I am going to put this into practice right away and report to you in a week.

Rupinder reported back in 6 weeks. She had been exercising regularly and felt fresh till about lunchtime. She would take a 15-minute nap, or let's call it siesta, and then, she was in mint form for the rest of the day.

Prior to the siesta, lunch is also a good opportunity to spend quality time with family and friends, which would otherwise have to take place in the evening or over the weekends. Taking a nap during the middle of the day means that many people are refreshed for the evening. It can also take pressure away from nocturnal sleep, where most people feel as if they have to sleep during this time. This is something that we should all consider, if appropriate, and we are able to do so. As they say, 'Don't knock it until you have tried it.' If a short nap at some point during the day works for you, then try and stick with it. If it supports your health and well-being, promotes productivity, and has a positive impact on your life, then who says that you cannot do it!

At all times, we need to think of the relationship between movement, sleep, the mind and nutrition, and not just in isolation. The other three almost always play a role in sleep disorders. But like most doctors, even sleep experts can easily miss out on those connections.

Throughout his early teenage years, Darren suffered from a sleep disorder following a viral infection. Sometimes known as 'post-viral fatigue', it can last for many months and even years, and develop into chronic fatigue syndrome. The causes for these types of disorders are not known and there aren't too many (if any) effective treatments. In Darren's case, he eventually 'grew' out of it, after accepting that if he was tired, he just needed to get rest and sleep. The one thing that he realized was that it was important to balance exercise and rest, as exercise in itself, if done properly, can actually make you feel energized, rather than fatigued. Paul Chek, a holistic health practitioner from the US, has coined the phrase to 'work in'. Rather than 'working out', where you burn energy, the idea of 'working in' is that you can actually get energized from performing exercise if done in the right way. Yoga and tai chi also have this as a foundation, which is why so many people do these activities as meditation.

Earlier, we mentioned about sleep quantity and quality. Let us delve deeper into it. There are a few basic things that we should all be doing to promote quality and quantity of sleep. The concept is called 'sleep hygiene'. This refers to the environment and behaviours that we engage in prior to sleeping. If either of these are not conducive to sleeping, then it can have a huge impact on our ability to sleep and also the quality of sleep that we get.

Early to Bed or Late?

As covered earlier, our ancestors slept according to nature. At sunset, they got ready to sleep and at sunrise, they got up. But as things changed, we all sleep and wake up at different times.

In the modern world, humans broadly fall into two basic categories when it comes to waking up in the morning—we are either 'morning' people or not! For some people, waking up early in the morning is very natural and they feel refreshed from a night's sleep. Other people struggle to wake up in the morning and perpetually hit the 'snooze' button on their alarm (if they have one, or indeed use their phone!). Such people often struggle to wake up and get the day started, only feeling fully awake and energized later into the day (and sometimes, not at all). This is other than the folks in whose case not getting up fresh in the morning can be a symptom of depression or other psychological conditions.

These types of waking behaviours have led to classification of people into 'a.m.ers' or 'p.m.ers', or 'larks' and 'owls' respectively. In scientific terms, we are considered to be a certain 'chronotype'. Chrono means time. In essence, our chronotype is determined by our underlying circadian rhythm, which is reflected in our sleep-wake patterns. You will notice that children have different sleep patterns. This can be genetic but also influenced by other factors—the environment, food, exercise, and many other factors. Modern society has forced us into one single chronotype, where we are all expected to wake at a certain time to be ready for school, work, etc. This pattern does not suit 'p.m.ers', as it means that they have to wake up early when their body and mind are not ready to do so. This can have a significant impact on people's lives where they constantly feel tired. The sad reality is that unless they begin to recognize their chronotype and make sleep and wake adjustments accordingly, they will never feel refreshed. For some people, this might mean changing jobs, so they can work in a job where they have more flexibility on start and finish time. Probably, 'work from home' courtesy COVID-19 has been a blessing in disguise for such people.

But there can be benefits in trying to influence your chronotype as well. Scientific studies have shown that 'p.m.ers' may have worse cardiac function compared to 'a.m.ers'. It has also been shown that most people are able to cope with stress a lot better early in the morning than later in the day, with 'a.m.ers' also being deemed to be happier.

The notion of chronotype does not just relate to waking times or patterns, but also to sleep. Knowing when to go to sleep seems like a very simple thing—you go to sleep when you feel tired. Unfortunately, modern society has, yet again, disrupted natural patterns of sleeping, where many people feel pushed into sleeping at certain times. For most people across the world, this will be between the hours of 10 p.m. and 12 a.m. In reality, this may be too early for some people and too late for others. This causes a disruption in the natural circadian rhythm which will have an impact on whether someone feels refreshed in the morning or not. The simple message is that you should sleep when you are tired and not when you think it is an 'acceptable' time to sleep. We are suggesting you sleep sooner, rather than later.

Sleep Alarm

Most of us only use an alarm to get up from sleep, but somehow, we take it for granted that we will sleep on time without being reminded. This might sound contradictory to the earlier advice of changing sleep times according to natural light, but it's not.

On a day-to-day basis, it helps to have the discipline to go to sleep and get up around the same time every day, weekday or weekend. It will help improve the quality and quantity of your sleep. As Dr Matthew Walker, professor, neuroscience, University of California, Berkeley, puts it, 'Deep within your brain, you have a massive 24-hour clock. It expects regularity, and works best under conditions of regularity, including the control of your sleep-wake schedule. Many of us use an alarm to wake up, but very few of us use a "to-bed" alarm. That's something that could be helpful.'[10]

'Men who sleep less than 5 hours a night have significantly smaller testicles than those who sleep 7 hours or more.' This fun fact shared by Dr Walker should get you to bed right away.[11] But lying in bed is not automatically equated to sleeping! Tossing and turning don't count.

Similar to men who sleep less and think they are 'Superman', women who sleep less think of themselves as no less than 'Wonder Woman'. Probably in women's case it's more to do with society. They are expected not only to have a professional life but also to do all the household chores while keeping the family together. As many as 90 per cent women are unaware that they suffer from sleep apnea,[12] which wreaks havoc in their lives. It's possibly because they have different symptoms than men do. While men snore, women tend to report excessive fatigue, sleepiness throughout the day, and mood or concentration lapses. They end up being misdiagnosed with depression or anxiety, and then are put on all kinds of drugs, when all they need is to sleep.

We also know that men who are sloppy, inactive and non-sporty tend to be sloppy everywhere. They have a higher desire for action in bed but don't last long, i.e., only if they are able to get started at all. Lack of sleep will affect the libido of women too, so we all need to ensure we are fully rested.

But if you are optimally active, you will be active in bed too, truly becoming an endurance athlete, before you literally hit the sack.

Having an alarm in place to plan your sleep is important, but it is not limited to just sleep time but working backwards and preparing to sleep too. Sleep isn't like a switch; we need to prepare for it. It's important to plan the timing of your dinner, coffee, alcohol and exercise, and change bedroom temperature, noise and light accordingly.

You should plan it in such a way that you must have had your dinner at least 2 to 3 hours before sleep. Some of us like to have a bedtime snack, but it is a bad idea. Also, having spicy dinner disturbs your sleep, so if you have to have a spicy meal, let it be lunch rather than dinner.

When it comes to alcohol, socially, it is associated with the night. But that, yet again, is doing no favours to your quality of sleep. Alcohol does make us drowsy, more so when we've had a bit more, but it doesn't let one go into deep sleep, leading to more disturbed sleep. For that reason, it is advisable not to have liquor in the last 4 hours before sleep.

For those of us who can't function without coffee, we need to relook at how you function because coffee consumption too close to sleep time is doing you no favours. On one hand, you have coffee to focus on your work, but when coffee comes in the way of the quality of your sleep and then you aren't rested enough for the next day, it's actually starting to come in the way of quality of your work time too. It is advisable to have your last cup of coffee no later than 6 hours before your planned sleep time.

Both coffee and alcohol inhibit your rapid eye movement (REM) sleep. That's when you recover and dream, which is essential for preparing you for the next day. That's when good-quality sleep comes along.

Exercising at the appropriate time of the day is also an important consideration, so as not to disturb your sleep patterns. Exercise also plays an important role in supporting sleep, which is still overlooked by many health professionals. Regular exercise can promote many of the physiological and psychological processes that support sleep, which can be seen with 30 minutes of regular exercise daily. However, when you exercise during a 24 hour-period can also affect the quality of sleep. Some people like to exercise first thing in the morning, prior to going to work or other activities for the day. Although this is a great start to the day, the body does take some time to get out of 'sleep mode' and into 'exercise mode', so the type of exercise undertaken should be carefully considered. For example, it would not be advisable to do heavy resistance immediately upon waking, as this may put you at risk of injury. Lower-intensity exercise such as a walk or light run can be used to get your body ready for more intense exercise.

Likewise, exercising late at night prior to sleeping can seriously disturb sleep. Exercise is a stress for the body (a good one though!), so there needs to be time for the body (and mind) to rest and recover and get ready for sleeping. In particular, the nervous system needs a chance to 'calm down' following exercise, so that you are in a state that can allow you to sleep. Exercising too close to sleeping will disrupt your circadian rhythm and, therefore, you should avoid exercising no less than 2 hours before you plan to sleep. An after-dinner stroll for 10–15 minutes is a good idea, but not a hard workout.

We should give enough respect and importance to sleep, because, as Dr Srivastava highlighted, one-third of our sleep time actually controls two-thirds of our wakeful time.[13] Like we prepare ourselves for the day after getting up in the morning, we should do the same when we are getting ready to sleep. Start with a shower or washing your face and then get into comfortable and loose sleeping clothes. This ritual starts preparing your mind for sleep. Bedclothes should ideally be made from natural material, which is not too heavy and allows for body temperature to be regulated. The same applies for bedcovers and bed sheets. Change them every week, if not more often, so that they are welcoming and cosy.

The purpose of a mattress is to allow the body to rest in a 'natural' position when sleeping, supporting the curvature of the spine and positions of the limbs. If a mattress is too soft, the body will not support itself and therefore, it will rest or move into a position that puts strain on the joints, making you sink into the mattress. Likewise, if a mattress is too hard, the body will not be able to rest in a suitable position. 'Memory foam' mattresses have become popular in recent years, having initially been developed as part of a research programme for space flight. Manufacturers report that these mattresses 'remember' your sleeping position and therefore, support the needs of your body. Unfortunately, if the original sleeping position is not suitable, then the mattress will remember the 'wrong' position. Technology has improved, but the best mattresses are those with natural material and pocket springs. A simple tip is to look for a mattress that is soft for the top inch to address your body contours, but hard below such that you don't sink in.

The same goes for pillows and bedclothes. Most of us use the pillow incorrectly. It is not meant only for the head and if the pillow is too thick or too thin, it backfires. A pillow should support the curvature of the neck so that the head is supported properly. Whether sleeping on your back or your side, most people rest their head on a pillow with no support under the neck. This can put unnecessary strain on the neck and lead to discomfort and pain. One simple solution is to roll up a towel and position it inside the pillowcase so that the neck is supported.

Along with preparing your body and bed for sleep, you need to plan your bedroom for the same too, more so during the last 1 hour before sleep. To begin with, your bedroom is meant for sleep and making love. This is one place that should not be a multipurpose room.

This may be difficult for people with restricted living space, but there should certainly be a 'divide' between areas of other activity and sleeping. This helps the body recognize the environment for sleep and helps to prepare accordingly. The simple act of getting the room ready for sleeping i.e., making sure the bed is made, etc., will also help when it is time to go to sleep.

It is tempting to watch TV, play video games, browse on smartphones, etc., in the bedroom, but these habits are not conducive to supporting sleep. In fact, some behaviours will do the exact opposite. Reading books, meditating, or listening to calming music can help with sleep, but it is important not to become reliant on such things in the long term unless they are something that can be sustained.

As mentioned earlier, the sleep of our ancestors used to be regulated by natural light. Then came along the light bulb and changed everything. We need darkness to sleep optimally, but in this artificially 24/7 lit world, as Dr Walker says, 'We are a dark deprived society.'[14] We may have overcorrected in our quest for light.

At least 2 hours before you sleep, definitely the last 1 hour, should be a 'screen-free zone' especially smartphones, tablets, laptops, desktops and even televisions. This can be difficult when we are so attached to devices now, but technology 'detoxes' can be healthy for the mind and relationships with friends and family. All artificial lights emit what is known as 'blue light'. This is part of the spectrum of light that is absorbed by our eyes and disrupts the signal required for melatonin to be released which helps in recovery. Over time, it can also damage the eye, whereas ultraviolet (UV) light from the sun can be restorative. In the last few years, it has become relatively popular to use blue light blocking glasses, or filters for TVs, laptops, and smartphones, to prevent disruption to sleep. This is often used to extend the working day so that people can work late into the night.

Dim down half the lights in your house. You'll be quite surprised at how sleepy that can make you feel. Using eye masks and blackout curtains can help create an even better environment to sleep well.

Your bedroom temperature is important, something we don't pay enough attention to. Pause here for a moment and just think as to when you feel like not getting out of bed? Is it in summers or winters?

That answer tells you what temperature your body likes when it comes to sleep. Our brain and body like to lower their temperature to initiate sleep. Having the room temperature set to a little colder than you normally have is helpful for sleep. Your bedroom temperature should be 17–18 degrees Celsius for at least 30 minutes before your planned bedtime.

Want to, But Can't

'If you have been trying to sleep and it's been 25–30 minutes or if you have woken up and can't get back to sleep, get out of bed (go to a different room) and go do something different,' says Dr Walker.[15] As much as your brain associates your bed with going to sleep, it also associates the same bed with waking up. It doesn't help tossing around in bed struggling to sleep. Only come back to bed when you are sleepy. But when you are sleepy, sleep. Then don't do other things. 'Gradually, your brain will learn that your bed is a place for sound and consistent sleep.'[16]

You can't just lie down and expect sleep to just come right away. At least that's not how it works for most. It isn't a switch that you can just turn off. According to Dr Walker, 'Sleep is like landing a plane.' You need to land the plane on the runway after which it slows down before coming to a complete halt. In this case, your brain. 'It takes time for your brain to gradually descend down on to the firm bedrock of good sleep. In the last half an hour to an hour, disengage from your computer and your phone, and try to do something relaxing. Find out whatever works for you, and when you have found it, stick to that routine.' So strictly avoid helicopter landing.

Avoid Night Shifts

Some people work in industries that require working in night shifts. This can have a profound effect on sleep quality and there can also be potential long-term health consequences if well-being is not managed. Night shift workers age faster than their peers not doing night shifts.

Poor sleep leads to increased appetite and a preference for calorie-dense, high-carbohydrate foods. This happens by reducing leptin, a hormone that tells the brain that there is no need for any more food. Also, ghrelin, a hormone responsible for triggering hunger, is increased. The desire to eat healthy foods like fruit, vegetables and dairy products is reduced and there is a craving for junk foods like candy and cookies. Poor sleep, whether because of night shifts or otherwise, has contributed majorly to increase in insulin resistance, type 2 diabetes and obesity.

Night shift patterns with regards to exercise, nutrition and sleep are a very personal thing. Some people like to 'mirror' their normal daytime activities at night, whilst others completely change their activities during their night working patterns. The simple advice would be that exercise and *MoveMint* should form a big part of your daily activity, even when working night shifts. This may mean waking up earlier prior to the shift to do some exercise or exercising when you return home before taking rest. Where possible, *MoveMint* should be incorporated into your work tasks. This can include breaking up your sitting time, taking regular walks, and doing some of the basic bodyweight exercises we cover in this book.

In summary, we all need to get more 'in tune' with sleeping, getting back to the basics (and nature) about what is going to help us get the rest and recovery we need.

Sleep Disorders

Like in all other lifestyle diseases, changing one's lifestyle and becoming more physically active helps address lifestyle and infectious diseases, and improves your quality of life. But there is still a role for medical attention. Similarly, if you have a sleep disorder or insomnia, these tips will help most but there might be a need to consult your doctor or a sleep specialist.

7

MoveMint Nutrition

It is no mistake that 'mint' is part of the phrase coined by us, *MoveMint Medicine*. Including a natural herb used in many recipes all over the world helps us emphasize the importance of nutrition. More than 3000 years ago, Greeks used to rub mint on their arms believing it would make them stronger.[1]

This ancient belief is not backed by scientific proof but another one has stood the test of time. Hippocrates, the Greek physician and philosopher, is claimed to have once said, 'Let food be thy medicine, and let medicine be thy food', although this is contested.[2] For thousands of years, natural remedies and foodstuffs were used as preventative and treatment medicines before the advent of the pharmaceutical industry. Although the use of pharmaceuticals in modern medicine has saved millions, if not billions, of lives over the past few decades, basic knowledge about the benefits and quality of food has somehow faded into obscurity.

Unfortunately, doctors and many healthcare professionals do not study nutrition when they are in training or at least not to the extent that they should. There might be a few lectures dotted throughout the years, but these are largely related to the biochemistry and digestion of food, rather than food and nutrition *per se*. In fact, many would argue that even the curriculum of some nutritionist and dietitian courses does not cover the information that is necessary to empower individuals to transform their health. Not only is nutrition understudied, but it is also not integrated into medicine. Consequently, it does not form a key part of any speciality. Whether it is applied in oncology, orthopaedics, obstetrics, or any other discipline, food and nutrition have a key role to play.

The biggest issue with poor food choices is that the effects are not felt or seen immediately. Bad dietary habits can be maintained for years before any negative impact on health is actually visible. However, consuming 'bad' food over a long period of time will cause health issues and contribute to a number of non-communicable diseases. The most prevalent of these diseases across the world is obesity. Excess body fat can lead to chronic insulin resistance (insulin not working as it should) and inflammation, ultimately contributing towards the development of diseases such as type 2 diabetes, cardiovascular diseases, cancer and musculoskeletal diseases.

The obesity situation in India has been termed by Dr Phil Maffetone as the 'overfat pandemic',[3] as it has now reached pandemic proportions. It is a crisis on an enormous stage and one that the country cannot possibly bear—the economic and societal impact of such a situation on a country the size of India can bring it to its knees. Such a crisis can neither be solved by doctors and other healthcare professionals, nor by the introduction of certain policies by the government. It can only be solved by changes that individuals make to their eating habits and by leading a *MoveMint* lifestyle.

From 2010 to 2040, when the Indian population is estimated to increase by 30 per cent, the number of obese persons is estimated to triple—a 300 per cent increase.[4] Every third person will be overweight and every tenth person obese. The biggest change is going to be in the elderly and the rural population, as they move towards 'westernized' dietary habits. To change that and have a healthier quality of life, for ourselves and our loved ones, they need to make basic changes *today*.

We are often told that 'we are what we eat', referring to the fact that our health is a reflection of what we eat. Although there is some truth to this, it would be more accurate to say that 'you are what you eat eats', referring to the quality of soil that 'feeds' the fruit and vegetables we eat or the quality of food and pasture that animals we consume eat. With this in mind, whenever possible, we should try and eat food that is grown and raised in the best environment imaginable. If it is possible to buy certified organic food, then that would be a good option. If this is not a feasible choice, we should try to buy the best quality of food available. This could mean looking to buy directly from farmers or farmers' markets rather than going to a supermarket. When buying dairy or meat products, it is advised to go for animals raised in a free-range environment rather than in a confined 'battery' environment that is the norm with intensive farming. Just like humans, animals are also born to move. So, the quality of milk or meat that comes from animals is also dependent on the amount that they have exercised.

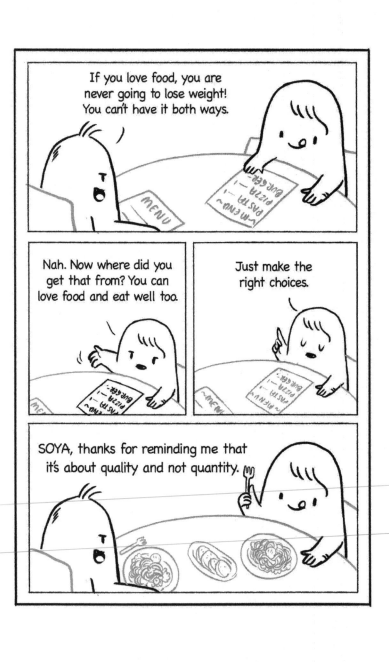

Growing food is something that many people across the world already do. However, for most of us, with busy working and personal lives, a majority of our food is purchased from supermarkets. Growing food not only ensures that the quality of the soil and the process of growing itself is in our own hands, but it also brings us 'closer' to our food and provides a sense of achievement and accomplishment. For children, being involved in the process of growing food provides us with an opportunity to educate them about food and its importance in supporting health throughout life. In our opinion, most children today are not familiar with where their food comes from. For them, it is either the supermarket or the delivery person who may have dropped it off. Many children cannot even recall the names of the most widely consumed vegetables, so involving them in growing and cooking food is something that should be widely encouraged. We highly recommend that you start a small terrace garden or balcony farming.

We would also encourage you to prepare and cook your own food. Processed foods are more likely to have additives, preservatives and other unnecessary ingredients which ensure that the food looks and tastes good while lasting for a long time on the shelf. Single-ingredient foods that can be put together as meals ensure that we have control over the food we eat. We also have control over what we add in terms of flavour enhancement—herbs, spices, etc.

There have been cases in recent times where children have been so malnourished due to overconsumption of fast food that they have become blind as a result of the lack of key vitamins. Food should not just be seen as something to satisfy one's hunger and cravings, but as medicine to fuel one's health. Just like we need to listen to our body about how much to move, we also need to be more in tune with the need for food.

Unfortunately, the highly processed nature and excessive sugar in a lot of food available to us has completely changed our instincts and behaviour with food. There have been some fascinating studies that look at the response of the reward centres in the brain when we consume food with high sugar. Sugar can almost act like an addictive substance (drug), activating the parts of our brain that trigger the desire to eat more and more. Fizzy drinks are a classic example of this, whereby the amount of sugar, colouring agents and other additive substances contribute to a 'potion' that is highly addictive. These types of drinks have finally started to receive over the years the bad press they deserve, leading some countries such as the UK to develop a 'sugar tax'.[5] Unfortunately, like many other health policies, this does not address the issue at the individual level. People are prepared to pay extra money to get their fizzy drinks. Shockingly, it is not just this industry that needs attention in this area. The hot drinks industry, which is growing at a phenomenal rate worldwide, is also using sugar and additives to get its customers addicted to its drinks. In the run-up to Christmas in 2021, UK coffee shop chains launched 'festive' drinks containing up to 63 grams of sugar.[6] That is 24 grams more than the amount of sugar found in a 330-ml can of cola!

Excessive intake of sugar can have a huge implication for our short-term as well as long-term health, affecting everything, from psychology and mental health to sleep and activity levels.

* * *

Nutrition and the state of one's diet, can have a profound effect on health and well-being. However, it may not be obvious until we do something about it. This was certainly the case for Ajay Mehra (*name changed*).

Ajay had been struggling with sleep. He and his wife, Pooja (*name changed*), went to see Dr Nidhi Dhawan, an ear-nose-throat (ENT) expert, for a consultation. He came into the room, sat down, put his head on the table, and just dozed off, snoring away to glory. Ajay was a 'healthy' 118-kg man. Pooja pointed out that Ajay could 'happily' go to sleep anywhere, any time!

Ajay woke up suddenly and said, 'Please operate on my nose.' When Dr Dhawan inquired why, he said that he was unable to breathe properly. When Dr Dhawan examined him, she found no problems in his nose. It was obvious that obesity was his problem. So, Dr Dhawan asked Ajay if he had done anything about his weight. Ajay told her that he tried everything but nothing seemed to work. 'Right now, I'm in a very desperate situation. I live on the fifth floor and the window faces the road. So, the other day, I was on the phone, talking to someone. I try to be active, so I was walking while talking on the phone. I walked towards the open window and the next thing I knew—I was hanging out of the window, with my arms over the window. I had just dozed off. My wife had to drag me back by my feet, else I would have fallen to my death. That day, we realized that I could go to sleep anywhere, any time, and while doing anything. It could be while standing, sitting, driving, etc. I am like this because I am unable to sleep at night. Please operate my nose.'

Dr Dhawan bluntly told him that looking at the current level of his physical fitness, he wouldn't even pass anesthesia fitness, i.e., get a go-ahead from an anesthesiologist for surgery.

'For a month, let's work on your weight,' she suggested. However, Ajay was adamant that nothing worked for him and he had tried everything under the sun. Dr Dhawan told him, 'Let's try out a very simple thing daily. When you get up in the morning and before you go back to sleep at night— just twice a day—drink a glass of warm water, followed by climbing stairs as slow or as fast as you like, continuously for 5 minutes. Just don't stop. Climb up and then go down the stairs. The only other thing I want you to do is, don't change anything in your diet. Have as many rotis as you want and as much ghee as you want but cut added sugar totally. No sugar at all. You don't need to do anything else. Just these two things.'

A month later, a thin man strolled into Dr Dhawan's consultation room and sat down right across from her. She didn't know him and found it awkward as she was eagerly waiting for Ajay. This stranger pushed a sheet of paper towards Dr Dhawan. She recognized it immediately. It was her letterhead with a prescription for Ajay. Dr Dhawan was confused. This man followed it up with a very peculiar, 'Doctor sahab', which Dr Dhawan found sounded very familiar. She simply couldn't believe it. It was Ajay! He had lost 20 kg in a month.

Ajay told her that he would forever be indebted to her as she had changed his life. He no longer felt the need for any surgery, was able to focus on his work and remained attentive towards his family too.

Later, Dr Dhawan confided in us. 'I knew that walking up and down the stairs combined with cutting down sugar helps, but I had personally never tried it for a month. I did what I had prescribed to Ajay. Lo and behold, I lost 7 kg in

1 month with just 5 minutes of stairs and zero sugar intake. Sometimes, it takes very little to turn the switch. It's not rocket science; it is very simple. But it is about consistency. I have never seen such a drastic result with such basic advice. We all see such changes happening with simple advice, but this was really something. For Ajay, this effort of going up and down the stairs was huge. And cutting out sugar totally was extreme but he just followed the instructions to a tee, one step and day at a time.'

Dr Dhawan told Ajay, 'There is no happy new year or happy birthday. Going forward, you will not miss a day. It is not something you do for just 1 month, it's a lifelong commitment to yourself. Please just be at it.'

Dr Dhawan shared with us, 'Whether children or adults, those who have excessive screen time with almost no physical activity, have a bit of extra weight around their waist and tend to have more breathing problems, more snoring at night and sinus issues. They also have a greater deficiency of vitamin D. My observation is that those who are active don't need any or as many supplements as sedentary folks. If you demand it from the body, it works and it seeks it out itself. If not, it's dependent on external supplements.'

* * *

Even though initially, as a species, we needed food to stay alive, with the abundance of food we have, there is no longer a need to go hunt and find food. But even today, pretty much for all of us, there is a desire to eat food that tastes good. We begin rewarding ourselves with food, starting with candies and chocolates, from childhood which carries on throughout our lives.

There are a number of reasons why we have become 'detuned' to what we actually need as food. The abundance and availability of food means that we have access to whatever food we desire or crave, whenever we want it. The commercial food industry has also conditioned us to believe that we need three meals per day. This might be changing with the development of some diet approaches discussed further below. But most of us eat three 'square' meals per day. What foods are consumed in each of these meals has also mostly been driven by the food industry, although there are differences across the world and in different cultures. For example, for many people across the world, a 'breakfast' will include the consumption of some form of cereal. Such cereals are almost always high in sugar and often have to be fortified with vitamins to ensure that they have adequate nutritional value. Such cereals may be convenient as a quick and accessible breakfast, but we should be mindful of what we actually need.

The notion of 'mindful' or 'intuitive' eating is exactly as it suggests. We should be more aware of what we need to be eating at a particular time. For example, it is not wise to consume a large meal immediately prior to exercising. Likewise, if you have completed an exercise session, it would not make sense to eat more than 2–3 hours later. Our bodies have adapted to our behavioural patterns with food. So when we think we are 'hungry', it could actually be related to our regular pattern of eating rather than our actual physiological hunger. As has been mentioned a number of times, food is fuel, so it is quite acceptable to go for longer periods without food if you are not exercising.

Food provides energy for exercise and movement. So, the recommendation would be to ensure you eat no less than 2 hours before you exercise. Having said this, it is possible to exercise 'fasted', with some scientific studies showing that this may be beneficial for how the body adapts. Many people now look to well-marketed commercial foods, drinks and supplements to help performance when exercising. Examples include gels, energy drinks, isotonic drinks and protein bars. For the average person doing regular exercise, these are not needed at all. It can make a difference to elite performance—you may have seen athletes carrying bottles along during a major marathon. Another common question around food and drink during exercise is the amount of water that should be consumed. As long as you are adequately hydrated prior to exercising (if you pass a low volume of urine that is dark in colour, it means you are dehydrated and you need to drink more water), for most people there is no need to carry a water bottle. Only in very hot conditions or when exercising for prolonged periods, is there a need for water. Drinking water to stay hydrated is important, but you must listen to your body. There can be severe consequences if one drinks too much water—termed hyponatremia—where sodium concentrations in the blood drop to dangerously low levels.

One aspect of hydration that many people overlook is the necessity for electrolytes. These are minerals that help regulate the amount of water in certain areas of our body and ensure that water goes where it needs to. As such, electrolytes are fundamental to health but also help with performance during exercise. It would be recommended, particularly in hot environments, that a standard 'over the counter' rehydration salt should be consumed once during the day to support electrolyte levels.

Eating after exercise is also recommended as the body is more 'sensitive' to the absorption of nutrients following exercise. In fact, this can be a very useful tool in the treatment of diabetes, where exercise can promote the transport of glucose from the blood to the muscle without the need for insulin. When you consume food after exercise is not really important, but it would be advised to ensure that you are recovered and rested before consuming a large meal. Blood will travel to the muscles to provide oxygen and nutrients to them even when you have stopped exercising, to support recovery. If we start eating a large meal during this time, the body will want to 'divert' the blood to the gut to help with digestion.

Being mindful of the requirements for food after we exercise is also important. For example, following a long run, it is necessary to have a meal containing some carbohydrates such as rotis, pasta, rice, etc. If you have just completed a strength training session or a fast or long run, it is important to ensure that you consume sufficient proteins in meals that follow. Such an approach may seem simple, but many people forget or overlook these basic principles.

The amount (volume) of food that we eat has also increased in recent years as the food that we consume is not satisfying. Although some foods are now more calorie dense, since they do not provide adequate nutritional value, the body does not get the signal to stop eating. Eating behaviours such as fast eating, the use (or not) of cutlery or other utensils, can also affect how much we eat and how satisfied we feel. The hunger response is mainly hormonal which means that it can take a while for the hormones to be activated/deactivated to send the signal to the brain and tell us that we are full. For this reason, it is recommended that you stop eating when you feel that you are 75–80 per cent full. Some recent studies have found that the size of the spoon can relate to the amount of food we eat. A smaller spoon means that we eat slower and, therefore, the feeling of fullness will be experienced sooner. Hence, we eat less.

Eating meals together has been a 'social event' since the birth of the human race. Unfortunately, in modern society, people are getting food 'on the go' or eating separately according to their own schedule. This has had some negative impacts on eating habits too, as people generally eat faster on their own and are unlikely to talk to anyone while eating. Preparing fresh and quality meals for one person or a limited number of people is also seen as difficult and time-consuming. So, processed meals are often used for convenience. Social or family pressures of eating are also taken away when eating on your own—this can be seen as a positive thing in some circumstances, where there can be a pressure to eat more food from friends or family. For others, eating in a social setting can stop them from 'binging' and eating too much, while eating alone means that they are likely to consume more food, perhaps of a poor nutritional quality. We recommend that as much as you can, eat your meals as a family.

For some individuals, food can cause issues. It stretches from minor discomfort related to digestion to serious adverse reactions (anaphylaxis) requiring immediate intervention and treatment. Such conditions are becoming more prevalent, with some scientists and doctors linking them to the poor quality of food available. Conditions such as irritable bowel syndrome (IBS) and other gastrointestinal disorders can get exacerbated due to consumption of certain foods which lead to chronic low-grade inflammation. An example of this is digestive discomfort (sometimes leading to IBS) caused by lactose intolerance. Lactose is the sugar found in milk which must be broken down in the small intestine so that it can be absorbed. As humans, we have an enzyme which is required to break down lactose called 'lactase'. It is primarily there to support us in the early stages of development when we are being breastfed. Being the species that we are, we also consume animal-derived dairy products which too contain lactose. Although the exact mechanism for lactose intolerance is not known, for many, it is related to the ability of our body to produce sufficient amounts of lactase. If the cells of the small intestine that produce lactase are inflamed (for one reason or another), the ability to produce lactase can be reduced.

When visiting India some years ago, Darren suffered from a case of Delhi belly. He had only passed briefly through Delhi on the way to Punjab! After a few days of gastrointestinal discomfort, he managed to recover but his digestion has never been the same. He is now very sensitive to dairy products and regularly takes them off his diet or significantly reduces the amount of dairy he consumes. It took many months to get 'in tune' with what was causing these issues and systematically avoiding dairy products over other food items. It is a very personal thing and something that many people go through, no matter what the food intolerance is. The most important thing to note is that we all need to be more aware of the food we are eating and how our body responds to it—both in the short term like bloating, fullness, fatigue, etc., but also in the long term like increase in weight, gastrointestinal issues, skin irritation, etc. Others have had similar experiences with grains. Such allergies and reactions are not looked into enough but have become common in today's society.

There is a very simple thing that can have an immediate and positive impact on our digestion. In our busy modern-day lives, we do not take the necessary time to sit down and eat our food properly. Most people eat a meal whilst doing something else—either watching TV or while being fixated on their other electronic devices. We also rush when eating and do not chew properly, resulting in what is called 'scoffing', i.e., eating your food far too quickly, without allowing time for your teeth to chew and break down your food.

Rajat's dad has some very important and profound advice when it comes to how we should eat our food. 'It takes almost no time to eat food, hours to make it and years to grow it. Slow down when eating food, cherish each bite and keep smiling.'

We need to remember that digestion starts even before food enters our mouth. By simply seeing and smelling food, our digestive system prepares to accept and digest food. Much of the digestive process also happens in the mouth—either through the mechanical action of breaking the food down with teeth or with the enzymes present there. The more time we take to chew food, the better it gets broken down and puts less stress on the stomach and the rest of the digestive system.

There are other considerations for nutrition including certain dietary preferences and also choices related to religious beliefs. Such things have to be respected, but it is important to be educated about the food choices you make. If there are certain restrictions in diet (e.g., meat or dairy), then there must be a wide variety of protein sources included that will provide sufficient protein and the range of amino acids. Most of our diets are very restricted, based on the foods that we are familiar with and what we are comfortable preparing and cooking. Variety is key to ensuring that we get a range of nutrients in our diet, particularly when there are certain restrictions on food. When it comes to vegetables and fruits, think about the colours in the rainbow, i.e., consume foods of different colours.

The 'No Diet' Diet

Every season, a new 'fad diet' crops up. This could range from vegan, Mediterranean, Atkins and paleo to ultra-low carb, ultra-low fat, Dukan, intermittent fasting, the zone diet, etc. Many people spend large parts of their lives jumping from one diet to the next, hoping to find that magical bullet that will help them get the body of their dreams. Nearly all diets will work to some extent for a short period of time and people will see changes within hours or days. However, in reality, there should not be a diet. We should all follow the 'no diet' diet, where we make permanent and sustainable changes to our eating habits.

Here is some 'food for thought'. We recommend reducing carbohydrate intake as most cultures promote its excessive intake. On the other hand, we would recommend increasing fat and protein intake. Even though Rajat is a vegetarian, when it comes to a well-balanced diet, he suggests that everyone follows a non-vegetarian diet (i.e., diet that contains meat and animal products). Being a pure non-vegetarian and consuming minimal vegetables and fruits is not advisable either. This does not mean being a carnivore and only eating meat but being more mindful about where your food (and particularly protein) is coming from. Proteins are the building blocks of your muscles and you need them to recover faster after strenuous workouts such as walking, running, cycling, swimming, strength training, etc. Proteins are also essential for all functions of the human body, so we must consider where we are getting them from. If you are unable to eat meat, ensure you have a wide range of vegetarian protein sources, such as dairy, pulses, legumes, etc. Fats have got a lot of bad publicity and are confused with fat in the body. They are important for you. In any case, women can endure pregnancy for 9 months because of higher fat content in their bodies when compared with men.

We should pick best practices from the diets that work for us. But definitely don't go for extreme diets as they can be detrimental.

Fasting has been a part of cultures like India for thousands of years, where people fast once a week. Although intermittent fasting has become popular in recent years, we all need to remember that we fast every single night. We do not wake up at night to eat. Before the invention of electricity, humans would eat only during certain times of the day such as the sunrise or the sunset, etc. This could mean extended periods of fasting, maybe up to 14 hours per day, with a break from 6 p.m. (dark) to 8 a.m. (light). Breakfast is called 'break-fast' for a reason; we are 'breaking' the 'fast'!

Another myth to bust is in the area of supplements, which are called exactly that for a reason. You only need to take them to supplement your regular food if something is missing from your usual meals. Don't let them be the main source of any nutrient.

There is also an argument on actually wanting or needing to lose any weight at all. As the saying goes, 'muscle weighs more than fat'. Fair enough, a kilogram of muscle will be as heavy as a kilogram of fat, but muscle is a lot denser than fat. Hence, a kilogram of muscle will take a lot less space than fat. With that consideration, what we should be promoting is body re-composition where fat is lost and muscle is gained. There will be circumstances where body weight will need to be reduced. There should be less focus on the weighing scale and more on the health and well-being outcomes of any diet. Remember, there is no ideal weight. As this book is titled *MoveMint Medicine*, it goes without saying that exercise and physical activity go hand in hand with any 'diet'. *MoveMint* can never outrun (or exercise) a bad diet. But a good diet will always need exercise to go alongside it for overall health and well-being.

* * *

There is another aspect to nutrition that is often overlooked. This is where psychology and movement overlap and knowledge of nutrition is simply not enough. Thirty-seven-year-old Shikha Pahwa,[7] who loves to run fast and long, shares her experience that a lot of younger and older folks alike can relate to.

> *Food is fuel, food is nutrition, food is a necessity etc etc., obvious facts. But for a very small percentage of people in the world, food is the enemy. Hard to believe, but true. It's called an Eating Disorder (Ed).*
>
> *There are no predetermined causes for Eating Disorder & It's not easily identifiable either, since the symptoms are not obvious & mostly well-hidden. Hiding feelings & lying about the effects are common with Eating Disorder. Having scraped through it myself, I know how it is.*
>
> *When I got into college, I got into this negative, self-critical phase, where my excess weight (which was actually*

just a tad over the recommended healthy weight) became the biggest problem in life. Unfortunately, it wasn't just a phase, & had probably built up slowly over time, & got triggered by something, I'm not sure. But these things definitely don't happen overnight. What I did to solve the "problem" was a combination of a crash diet & exercise. Having done neither of the two in my life, the effect showed pretty fast. Now the goal was weight loss, but how much? Because nothing seemed to be good enough. The more I lost, the more I still wanted to lose. Plus the fear of gaining it back made me quite paranoid.

When I talk about the fear of gaining weight, it is not just a random thought that crossed my mind once in a while. It was there every single day, every time I ate, every time I just looked at food. Can you imagine how many times that is? All the time. Not just that, there was also the guilt of eating anything slightly different from the "acceptable" non-fattening food list I had created in my mind. This also made me make excuses to get out of situations where I would have had to eat with others, whether it was family, friends or other social commitments. I felt horrible doing it, & I now believe I lost out on some "quality time", which I really regret, but the consequences of getting through it seemed worse at that time. The fear, the guilt & then the extra exercise to get over that guilt; it was a vicious cycle. This went on not for weeks, not months, but for many years; and still, I was never at peace. Such feelings, as I once read, are experienced by most people with Eating Disorder. In fact, the advanced symptoms could be potentially fatal, and I was lucky to have never reached that far. But still, the battle of 'me versus me' hurt me physically and broke me mentally. I had the will-power, a lot of it actually, but used it for the wrong reasons; and was never happy about it.

Somewhere during this time, two things happened. First, I accepted that I had a problem & second, I discovered running.

Someone with Eating Disorder has to go through a lot of stuff, but the person's family suffers just as much. Just to identify the problem for them is a big deal, since most people still aren't aware of this particular disorder, and after that knowing how to deal with it is a whole new level of testing patience. In my case, it was my sister who kept it together in the most unbelievable way. To be watching a family member do something so wrong to themselves and not saying anything is incredibly difficult. She did it for years, not because she didn't want to, but because she knew it was only going to make me aggressive. With constant perseverance, she convinced me that I needed to get better & subsequently, to see a therapist to talk about it. There was a lot of resistance on my part initially but I agreed, and surprisingly, it wasn't as bad as I had thought. In fact, it wasn't bad at all. It was a pleasant conversation with someone who wanted to listen and encourage. I had a couple of sessions like that in the following months. It didn't have an immediate effect on me but definitely contributed in some way.

Initially when I started exercising, it was only a walk-jog on the treadmill that I used to do and it went on for a few months. I hated it; a forced thing to do every day. Finally I just decided to find another form of exercise and so found an interest in aerobics classes. It was a high intensity exercise and also fun to do, the only problem was that the days there was no class or it got canceled or I couldn't make it, I would get really anxious. There were times when I had to move my work around or ask others to work around my time so that I didn't miss it, which was quite unreasonable on my part. While aerobics was great, it did get a bit irregular at times. The only other option for me then, was to go for a walk. Since it wasn't 'intense-enough', I tried a little jogging in between. After doing this a couple of times, I progressed to jogging a few kms, and running soon after. Someone once suggested participating in a half marathon during that time. First I laughed it off, but then decided to take up the challenge. Having never run more than seven kilometers at a stretch, I had serious doubts about finishing it. With about two months of regular running I took the distance up to 14 km. The only goal was to finish the race, and I did, with a decent timing. The experience was nothing less than an exciting journey and I was completely hooked. I had finally found something I was good at, after a very long time. Since then, running has become a major part of my life (for different reasons), with a desire to perform better every time.

Now here is the irony – indirectly, I stumbled upon running because of Eating Disorder. The desperation to exercise got me running, and then the drive to improvise is what started pulling me out of it. In some twisted way, should I be grateful for it? It is a fact that nutrition is the foundation of running, and I knew that for any improvement in terms of distance and speed, my diet wasn't going to work. It wasn't easy at all and it took some time, but I did accept and work on it. The process was slow and not in proportion to the intensity of my activities, but I did the best I could. So from half marathons to full marathons and now to ultra marathons, I'm still striving (but very close) to achieve that perfect balance.

Have I gotten rid of Eating Disorder? Almost, I would say. I know all the facts, or I would like to believe, about Eating Disorder and I try to do the right thing. But there is still that voice in my head that stops me at times. I ignore it most of the time, but not always. It took me ten years to start taking *back control of my life, the recovery road being harder than I had imagined. I am still on the same path, gradually moving forward, far far away from where I started. I lost out on a lot of things over the years but that won't happen any more.*

The same Shikha ran 212 km in 2019 at La Ultra in Ladakh when there was a whiteout and blizzard on two back-to-back nights on both Khardung La and Wari La mountain passes that are over 17,400 ft altitude, temperatures had dipped down to minus 10. She started off 2022 with a 10-km run at a pace of 4-minute-and-30-second per km.

There are many generic hints and tips that can be offered around nutrition, but it really is an individual and situation-specific thing. Weston A. Price was a Canadian dentist who toured the world with his wife in the 1920s and 1930s to examine the diets and health of native communities. In his famous book, *Nutrition and Physical Degeneration*, published in 1939, he described how dental and overall physical health was often determined by the nutrition that was available to people in their local environment.[8] The most striking observation presented in the book was that native people, eating native diets, rarely suffered from any non-communicable diseases which were rapidly increasing in the western world. In contrast, if any of these communities abandoned their native diet and adopted an industrial western diet, they soon became sick. In other words, if you eat what is local, both figuratively and literally, you will receive the nutrition *you* need. Unfortunately, in modern society, we have lost this basic sense of what food and nutrition we need.

We believe this forms a major part of the problem that is causing all of the ill health across India and the world.

We have 'forgotten' what we should be eating. Rather, we are consuming what is advertised to us believing it to be the right food. Our recommendation is that you should be getting back to your roots, eating what your ancestors would have been eating—fresh, locally farmed and sourced food, without industrial processing.

8

MSK: 'M'ake 'S'ure You 'K'now

One would have thought that stories from different cultures and religions, told and retold over centuries by elders, would have taught subsequent generations an immense lot about health and fitness. Even among the ones who have listened to such stories, a majority have top-heavy bodies bent forward like a gorilla and pencil-thin legs and feet of clay (i.e., too much upper body work in the gym, whilst forgetting about the legs). More importantly, they have failed to learn anything from these stories. But then again, common sense is a rare commodity. We happily repeat the same mistakes, as if hell-bent on trying to master imperfection.

Aches and pains in muscles, tendons, ligaments, joints and bones, especially the back and knees, are way too common today. Courtesy the sedentary lifestyle we lead, there is no discrimination with regard to the social strata, race, gender, age, religion or skin colour, education or geographical area. We are all in it together. It's compounded further by excessive usage, more so in the last two decades, of all kinds of gadgets like smartphones and laptops from early life. If you can't move

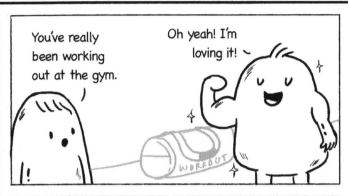

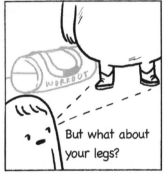

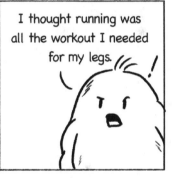

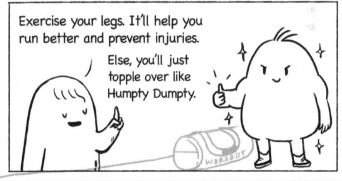

comfortably to do exercises of any kind, it's then a moot point to talk about other diseases or medical specialities. For that reason, we will focus on the 'neuro-musculoskeletal' system, a speciality which is somehow ignored by even the good doctors out there.

There are a lot of misconceptions and myths floating around about this topic, even in the medical fraternity. We'll break it down for you, touching on common conditions, so that you know better how to handle them. At the end of the day, our main objective is to motivate you to GOYA and get moving.

You might find it slightly repetitive from the breathing section, but it is what it is. After all, repetitive breathing keeps us alive. If only Duryodhan had taken a long, deep breath and thought once about what Krishna was suggesting since there must have been a good reason why his mother asked him to do what she did.[1] But then, if Duryodhan could ever think with a cool head, he wouldn't have been in the situation that he was. He wouldn't have been him. It's up to all of us if we can learn from his mistakes and make our lives any better.

Has your doctor told you that breathing plays an important role in the treatment of your neck, shoulder, back or knee pain? Please go back and read the section on breathing along with this if you had skipped it earlier.

As mentioned earlier, we are way more than just a bag of bones; definitely a lot more than the skeleton hanging in the closet/the hospital or a doctor's consultation room. If we were just the skeleton, what would be the difference between us and the ones permanently resting in graveyards? We are alive; we can think; we can breathe and we can move. Let's not act dead before we *are* dead.

Don't run, don't exercise, don't walk, don't do this, don't do that! Let's not be told to act dead by well-meaning doctors because, most of the time, unknowingly, they end up suggesting exactly that. And we blindly follow that poor advice. Excuse them for their well-intentioned folly. After all, the first patient doctors see, as medical students, is a cadaver. It teaches an immense lot, but it's past its expiry date and has lost the ability to think and move. We need to use our ability to think for ourselves and move. Never blindly follow anything, be it in medicine, politics or any other field.

When we look at the skeleton, in that skull, there is something missing—the brain. The organ that helps you think, besides managing a lot of other important functions. Let us think and use the organ whose optimal functioning is crucial to keep us alive and kicking. If we don't use it, we'll lose the capacity to use it. So, let's think; something that wasn't a strong point for Duryodhan.

As mentioned earlier, if the brain is the hard drive, the mind is the software. As often stated, your thoughts are a sum total of all your experiences. The mind's role is undermined in modern-day medicine. Not enough emphasis is placed on what you can think and feel. Sadly, it's only about what the doctor can physically see in front of them and more often than not, pick up a supposed injury using high-tech investigative tools such as MRIs and CT scans.

The brain continues as a spinal cord, a snake-like structure, that is protected by the spine. The spinal cord branches out into nerves, the way a river branches out into tributaries, that spread out across the body. Think of the brain as a central processing unit and the spinal cord and the nerves as electricity cables, supplying electricity to the whole body.

They also send and take messages from the brain to the rest of the body. The brain, the spinal cord and nerves play a big role in the musculoskeletal system, and in all the aches and pains you develop in all your joints, muscles, tendons, ligaments, etc., throughout the body.

Your body could be as good as a top-end car. As a matter of fact, it is a lot more sophisticated than that. If, in that car, we were to cut the main wires, the ignition will not work and the car won't start, leave alone move. The same goes for our bodies. However, the brain and the spinal cord are extremely delicate.

Whether it was nature or God, these have been taken care of pretty well. The brain resides in the skull, and our brains are a lot safer that way. As children, when we all fell a million times and hit our heads on the floor, if not for our skulls, just one fall would have killed us.

Then there is the spinal cord. From the base of the skull till the waist level, there are twenty-four bones or the vertebrae stacked one above the other. They are jigsaw-like and fit well on top of each other. The front part of each vertebra is oval shaped, with a cushion-like disc between consecutive vertebrae. Each of the vertebral bones has a hole in the back of the bone, such that when they are stacked on top of each other, they form a cylinder-like tube. This protects the snake-like spinal cord. The brain continues as the spinal cord in the safety of the spinal canal formed by the vertebrae stacked on top of each other.

The skull sits on the neck, also known as the cervical spine. These are seven vertebral bones stacked on top of each other (C1–C7). The neck further sits on the upper and middle back, i.e., thoracic spine, which are twelve in all (T1–T12).

The ribs are attached to the thoracic spine, discussed in detail under the breathing section. In the front, the ribs attach to a tie-like bone called the sternum. The lungs and the heart are caged within the ribs. The thoracic spine is further stacked on the lower back, i.e., lumbar spine, which are five vertebral bones (L1–L5).

The lumbar spine sits on the base of an inverted, flat, triangular-shaped bone called the sacrum, which is between the hip bones. Sacrum is made of five smaller fused bones (S1–S5). The pointed part of the sacrum has a bone attached to it called the coccyx, yet again comprising three to five fused bones. The coccyx is also known as the tail bone.

Both the sacrum and coccyx bear the weight of the rest of the twenty-four vertebral bones of the spine, with the skull at the very top. Like the chassis of a high-end car, the sacrum provides good stability without compromising on the comfort of a smooth drive throughout our lives. For this comfort, similar to shock absorbers in cars, between any two consecutive vertebrae, there are discs, providing cushioning.

When Darren was learning anatomy during his undergraduate degree, his tutor used to recite an amusing acronym to help him to remember the vertebrae.

crazy (cervical–seven)
tutors (thoracic–twelve)
love (lumbar–five)
sniffing (sacral–five)
coke (coccyx–four)

Whether the crazy tutors sniffed 'coke' or not, this is certainly a good way to remember the structure of the spine.

The spine is S-shaped when we look at it from the side. The neck is convex and the upper and middle back are concave to accommodate the heart and lungs. The lower back is convex, giving us a tall posture.

The tributary-like nerves go out from the spinal cord at each level, exiting from the location of discs. Often, back pain is attributed to discs wearing out or discs bulging into the spinal canal, irritating the exiting nerves. There are a few things that we need to understand. In girth, the spinal cord is one-third the size of the space in the spinal canal. It has enough room to move around. Even when a disc bulges into the spinal canal, while it reduces space for the spinal cord, the spinal cord, being the snake it is, just slips away. Like a slippery, slimy politician.

Another major reason attributed to most back pains is degenerative discs. We need to understand that we are degenerating from the moment we are born. MRIs are very sensitive investigations. Our doctor colleagues attribute anything they find on MRIs to the clinical presentation, without knowing a patient's background—whether it is family, physical activity, psychology, sleep, nutrition, the environment the patient lives in, the belief systems or what the patient aspires to be. Research studies have repeatedly demonstrated that after the age of thirty, most people, irrespective of whether they have back pain or not, have to some extent, changes that show disc degeneration and disc bulges.

You are treated by the almighty doctors in a white lab coat with a black tube around their necks as if you don't have the capability to think or move. Please don't let them do that to you. Wrong words uttered by the doctor can amplify your pain. Your stress and anxiety play a major role in back pain. In most long-term pains, the mind plays a far bigger role than our colleagues can even comprehend. Sadly, most of them are simply not trained to address it.

Just think! We were made to move. Rather, we moved as a sperm even before we were born. But most healthcare professionals pass a death sentence and tell you to become a vegetable for life, even before your expiry date. The value of *MoveMint* has been lost and even with all of the evidence and recommendations that are available now, most medical professionals shy away from prescribing *MoveMint*.

The twenty-four bones, seven in the neck, twelve in the upper and middle back and five in the lower back, are meant for movement at each level. To bend forwards and backwards, sideways and to rotate as well. But courtesy our current, modern sedentary lifestyle, especially while using smartphones and all other gadgets, makes them stiff. When we have the slightest pain, this fear of moving the spine is made worse by the advice given by our medical colleagues— complete bed rest and no movement of the back.

And we were made to think, so don't let anyone, no matter what title they hold and whatever number of random alphabets follow their name, tell you otherwise. Of course, do listen to them, but think for yourself. They could have seen thousands of patients like you. Even with their best intentions for you, they are still working with statistics. Maybe 90 per cent of people got better with a certain approach, but you need to remember that they are not you. Get yourself engaged in your management. How can these doctor colleagues of ours pass a judgement after only knowing you for a few minutes? You need to know that most causes and symptoms of back pain can be addressed if you take a proactive role, both physically and psychologically.

When the lower back is painful, as a protective response, the upper and middle back muscles go into a spasm. The analogy worth thinking about is that of a twenty-four-storey building, where the ground floor is like the feet of clay of the statue in King Nebuchadnezzar's dream. Even though they are the foundation, they are the weakest. The floors above, like the statue, are top-heavy. The fragile lower back is compromised even more as the top layers, in this case upper and middle back, keep getting stiffer.

This stiffness, caused because of long years of poor posture and muscle imbalances, worsened further by pain, leads to you taking even shallower breaths, both because of anxiety and because physically, the lungs do not have enough capacity to expand. Your twelve ribs on both sides are attached to the twelve thoracic vertebral bones of the upper and middle back, i.e., half of the bones of the spine that have good mobility. Stiffness around the thoracic spine leads to restriction of movement of the ribs. And these stiff ribs make the upper back even stiffer. It is a catch-22 situation.

Once we take long deep breaths, getting that rib cage to expand, moving the bucket handle-like ribs up and down, our upper and middle back becomes more supple and muscles around the neck and upper back relax too. This breaks the vicious cycle and puts less pressure on the lower back. The same holds true for upper back, neck and shoulder pains too.

X-rays and MRIs: Boon or Bane

The introduction of X-rays in medicine was a game changer. For the first time, without needing to cut it open, we could see inside the body. Then, MRI, took it to a whole new level, where we could even see the soft tissues, i.e., everything else besides the bones. This helped identify what the problem was. X-rays, MRIs and all other such investigative advancements have changed the way medicine is practised today. Earlier, there was a lot of guesswork, but also a lot more art than science. Today, keeping the patient's best interests in mind and, in our eagerness to practise evidence-based medicine, at the cutting edge of science, we have let go of the art of medicine. We are no longer treating patients, but are busy treating investigation reports, X-rays and MRIs. Most of the time, the findings on these high-tech investigations are coincidental and not the cause of the pain.

It does become a problem in a country like India where the public understanding of diagnostic tools is poor and the tests are widely available. There can often be misdiagnosis leading to courses of treatment that are not needed or cause further complications. Dr Raju Easwaran, a sports orthopaedic surgeon, says that getting an MRI is as easy as going into a supermarket to buy some groceries. He adds that in India today, you can get an MRI for a scratch on the back!

There is definitely a place for MRI in identifying potential causes of musculoskeletal conditions and pains (and we are not denying this!), but it should only be done to verify and complement a clinical diagnosis. Some doctors are so focused on identifying anatomical abnormalities or changes on MRI, that they miss out on the real underlying cause. There are doctors, including Dr Easwaran, who are now wise to this and are using MRI only as a tool alongside the clinical context, to see where the patient is heading. But such doctors are few and far between.

Getting Back to Fitness: Amit, Amit and Arvind

While interviewing doctors and other healthcare professionals for this book, we often found that they were active in school.[2] But then, in high school, they started focusing more on studies to get better marks to get into good colleges. That inactive lifestyle carried on in college, where priorities, understandably so, are very different. When they get into work life, the rat race begins and they still don't think about themselves. The same applies to all other professionals as doctors are just a subset of the society. They aren't different from non-medics.[3]

Amit Kshirsagar an ultra-runner and running coach from Hyderabad, had always been an avid sports lover since childhood. He represented his college in badminton and luckily, he used to play it regularly for a few years even after college. Even though Amit isn't a doctor, he is similar to most doctors and healthcare professionals, who, in spite of being sporty in school and college, had to drop a physically active lifestyle. From 70 kg in 2000 when he was diagnosed with hypothyroidism (underworking thyroid), he became 105 kg in no time, unrecognizable to himself, leave alone anyone else. In 2002, he was diagnosed with high blood pressure and was put on medicines for the same.

He moved to Hyderabad in 2008 and that was a game changer. He picked up badminton and squash but his excessive weight led to extreme lower back pain. That's when he decided that he had had enough. He started changing his lifestyle. In 2015, Amit started cycling, slowly building his endurance. He was able to complete about 10,000 km that year and did 200-km brevets (long distance cycling event). Soon, he started focusing more on running than cycling. He does strength training twice a week, a weakness of most runners, where this is very much overlooked. He has run numerous half, full and ultramarathons. He does recognize that exercise alone is not enough, so he restricts his sugar intake and does not consume junk food at all. Since then, his weight has been in control and he now weighs 79 kg. He managed to come off his blood pressure medicines in 2018, after being on them for over 16 years. It was only fitting that he received the most improved runner award that year during the 'Hyderabad Runners Awards' night. Now, he is spreading the magic by mentoring and coaching others for running. Amit sums up his journey really well.

'What started as a weight-loss goal ended up being a journey of discovery of self. Today I don't run to lose weight. I run because I enjoy it! I run because I get to meet old and new buddies who have become an extended family. I love chasing new goals and it's a fantastic feeling of taking my body to places it's never been.'

As much as the trigger for lifestyle change could be a health shock, but to carry on the discipline for life, we need these activities to be fun. As mentioned in Human Givens, one of the needs is to be worthy of helping others and yet another one is the need to belong to a tribe. Amit has stated both above.

Also, when doctors experience what patients go through, they start empathizing more and have a totally different perspective. They become friends and guides to their patients without even realizing how sports, exercise and running is changing them.

Dr Amit Srivastava, a dental surgeon and orthodontist from Delhi, had represented his secondary school in football, cricket, and even long jump. But, as it often happens, he had to quit his active lifestyle during his undergraduate and postgraduate studies.

In 2000, he had a life-changing experience that has given him a whole new perspective. Dr Srivastava met with a road accident during his postgraduation and fractured a bone in his mid-back (the T−12 vertebrae). The treating orthopaedic surgeons told him to look after himself and focus only on the medical profession and forget about being active in sports. Dr Srivastava didn't like it one bit and in 6 months, he was swimming. Soon after, he was running too. He wasn't able to run fast but could run slow for long distances. He was starting to rediscover his old fit self and started enjoying it. It was also satisfying to prove the doctors, who had asked him to give up on his active and fit lifestyle, wrong. Back then, there wasn't much of a running culture. He then started going to the gym and lifting weights. He had been told after his accident that he was not to lift more than 5 kg but here he was, bench-pressing his body weight! Over time, Dr Srivastava was bench-pressing double his body weight. The best part was that he kept the pace of getting back to fitness gradual. He is a sportsman for life, who follows a basic rule:

'The will to win means nothing without the will to prepare.'

And prepare he does. It was in 2013 that Dr Srivastava picked up road running and, for the first time, participated in the Delhi Half Marathon. The running bug had bit him. He has now run numerous half-marathons and eight full marathons.

He is now in top running shape and is capable of running a respectable full marathon (42.195 km) in under 3 hours, a feat amongst amateur runners.

> *'Even though I am a dental surgeon, over the years, after having seen my running pictures on social media, a lot of my patients have contacted me for their chronic diseases like diabetes, hypertension, cardiac conditions, and obesity. Imagine that! Asking a dentist for fitness advice. At times, I need to do the same for patients who come for dental issues but have other lifestyle issues like high blood sugar. As specialists, we are too focused on body parts or a particular procedure and forget that there is a whole human being that we need to address. But, my running has helped me appreciate that I am not seeing only a set of teeth. My results are a lot better and my clients like my holistic perspective. I've become more of a life coach for most of my patients and not only a dentist.'*

* * *

At times, Eureka moments happen to doctors when they go through their own experience. Dr Arvind Bhateja, a neurosurgeon, has himself been on a very personal journey with back pain and fitness. Being active in school, his studies took over his active life. Once he had passed his medical training, he was overweight and unhealthy. He took up running in 2003. But it was not until some years later, when he picked up a copy of the *Runner's World* magazine that he developed a passion for long distance and ultra-running. Soon after this, he suffered from a meniscus (cartilage) tear and decided to take up cycling. Graduating from a mountain bike to a road bike, he began training and competing in long-distance cycling events. Ironically, in 2014, while Dr Bhateja was participating in a cycling event, he developed severe back pain. He had to be transported more than 600 km in an ambulance for surgery for his injured disc. A year later, having faced physical challenges to recover and after convincing his family that it was the right thing to do, he was back on the bike and racing in events again. It was his passion and love for cycling that made him do this. Cycling was his thing. This is where he connected with his higher self. It was important to him more than most people could comprehend. This gave him a whole new perspective on why patients wanted to continue performing certain activities that he earlier thought were causing them pain or making their injuries worse. In 2018, he had a repeat injury and had to undergo another surgery. Despite both surgeries, he is still very active and cycles long distances. He continues to promote exercise to all of his patients. So much so that he tells his patients that 'the only answer to their back pain issues is exercise'.

The physical fitness, stamina and resilience that he developed from cycling has not only helped in his own practice (being able to withstand long days in the operation theatre), but it allowed him to have a personal perspective to share the benefits of exercise with his colleagues and patients.

Knees: Dr Anjali and Madhav

Dr Anjali Kumar is a gynaecologist, endoscopic surgeon, an expert in high-risk pregnancy diseases, an ex-Army officer a yoga teacher and the founder of 'Maitri', a digital platform on women's health. She got into fitness in a big way at the age of forty-five, i.e., a decade ago. Until then, she was fond of walking and trekking, but there was no set regime that she used to follow. Since she wasn't overweight and didn't suffer from chronic diseases like diabetes or hypertension, she assumed that she didn't need to be fitter. One fine day, she developed back pain with sharp shooting pain down one of the legs. That really shook her up. No one was able to give her an answer. She consulted the best doctors and got all kinds of investigations done. That was the worst part of it. All that came up was an old, shrivelled disc. Since she wasn't getting better, she was advised to undergo surgery. That's when she was introduced to yoga and her back pain became better.

As luck would have it, she had another injury in her knee, a meniscal tear. She was managing it conservatively but it wasn't getting much better. The orthopaedic surgeon told her that she needed surgery (arthroscopic meniscectomy). She trusted the doctor and agreed to it. Unfortunately, her pain worsened after the surgery. And that's when she met Rajat. Yoga played a major role in her recovery. Now she is able to manage most things, including long hours standing as a doctor. She does strength training three times a week and does yoga 6 days a week. During the lockdown, she was very happy doing yoga even twice a day on some days. She now tells her patients that everyone should pay attention to exercise.

'Exercise needs to be a very happy and long term sustainable activity for you. If you dread going to the gym in the morning, probably that's not the right kind of exercise. You need to find something that gives you a happy feeling. It could simply be dancing, swimming, a game of tennis, yoga or it could even be

gymming. Yoga worked for me, so I am sure that people can find
out what their happy exercise is.'

Then there is Madhav Kumar from a decade ago. The then twenty-four-year-old gym buff wanted to join the Indian Army after his MCom for as long as he could remember. His father, who was a politician, too was keen on Madhav joining the Army.

Madhav cleared his Service Selection Board (SSB) examination for the Indian Army. One fine day, while getting up from a squat position, he twisted his right knee. He didn't think much of it then, but when he came back home, his knee had ballooned to the size of a baseball though it didn't hurt much. Over the next few days, the swelling disappeared and he kept training. As backup, just in case he didn't make it to the army, he was training for the physical examination for the position of a sub-inspector in the Delhi Police. By the time he was done with various exercises and physical activities, there was a lot of pain in his right knee.

He showed his knee to a top sports surgeon in the city at a premier sports medicine centre. Based on an MRI, he was diagnosed as having a (medial) meniscal tear, a ligament that stabilizes the knee joint, reduces friction during movement and absorbs about one-third of the impact that the joint cartilage surface goes through. Effectively, menisci are very important for optimal usage of the knee, especially while doing intense physical activities. The surgeon recommended surgery for Madhav. Under normal circumstances, this could have worked well for him. But any surgical intervention would automatically disqualify him from joining the Officers

Training Academy (OTA) in Chennai, for which he was supposed to report in just over 3 weeks. In a month's time, he was expected to run 2.5 km in 9 minutes, followed by 25 km of extremely tough cross-country terrain in under 3 hours.

That is when he consulted Rajat. After a detailed musculoskeletal examination, Rajat was of the opinion that Madhav had a good chance of getting into the army and didn't need surgery. But for that, there was a need for intense rehabilitation. This ray of hope was all that Madhav needed and he latched on to it.

Madhav didn't find the exercises taxing enough but after 2 weeks of rehabilitation, he was feeling much better. He was not yet comfortable running, leave alone running fast enough. Rajat met him one morning in the park to show him how to run more efficiently. Madhav's stride length was reduced and he was shown how to use gravity in his favour. After all, gravity is a pretty strong force that actually keeps planets in their place, so there is no point fighting it. His upright, stiff posture was changed to tilting forwards from the heels. Madhav's limited ankle and hip movements were addressed too, reducing the load on the knees.

Average and poor runners try to run from their knees whereas good runners run from their hips. Keep your breathing easy and not laboured. Land your feet softly. You shouldn't be able to hear them.

How is it possible that Rajat was right about Madhav but no one had mentioned any of this before? Madhav wasn't convinced but didn't have anything to lose, so he played along.

Rajat told Madhav to just keep up with him while running, each step of the way, occasionally reminding him to relax his shoulders, keep a tall posture, shorten his stride with soft landing and to keep deep-controlled breathing on. Together, they ended up running 2.5 km in 8.47 minutes. Madhav was amazed at what he had just achieved. And there was no knee pain. That instilled his faith in the process and he stuck with it. Madhav cleared his physicals and excelled at the OTA.

In 2012, Madhav came to see Rajat, and 9 years later, there is no pain. He has actually forgotten that he ever had a knee issue. Madhav admitted that through these years, he has put his body through a lot more rigours, especially during his short service commission stint of 5 years in the army. He adds, 'I excelled in my commando course and ran 30 km and 40 km in record times. I still carry on running and those unassuming rehabilitation exercises are the ones that have helped me immensely.'

So, what about 'running is bad for your knees' that's been thrown at us all forever, not only by our loved ones but also by the doctors, the supposed experts at this? As soon as you understand how to get moving and apply some common sense, you can do magic. Going back to the basics is what worked for Madhav. And it'll work for you too.

When Surgery Is Needed?

Exercising, running and sports have massive physical and psychological benefits, but sometimes, injuries can come along either because of those activities or, at times, for some other reason. It becomes important to have some sort of a plan to get back to being active, rather than being headstrong and avoiding surgery, leading to a permanent injury.

At times, for whatever health condition, surgery is the only option. That doesn't mean you rush into surgeries. But if you have to have a surgery, then how do you get back to being your healthy self?

If you require surgery and wish to get back to any level of physical activity, be it for leisure, health or competition, it is important to consider a number of factors which will determine your rate of recovery and your long-term health.

As modifiable factors, your health and state of 'fitness' prior to surgery will affect recovery and rate of recovery. An example of this is the amount of muscle mass relative to fat mass, which is thought to be a determining factor for recovery in cartilage and many other orthopaedic surgeries, or even surgeries seemingly unrelated to muscle. It is therefore important to ensure that you maintain health and fitness prior to your operation—this may require adapting your training to avoid pain and further dysfunction. Transitioning to some form of non-weight-bearing exercise as part of your regime will help reduce excessive load on damaged tissues.

Dr Anant Joshi, one of the first movers in the field of sports medicine in India, way back in 1984, was a champion badminton player in his school and medical college days. When he moved to the US in 1982 to specialize in arthroscopy (keyhole surgeries of joints) in sports medicine, he switched to tennis, playing at a decently high level. He saw the top sportspeople of the country as he was the only specialist in the field.

It was in 1989 that he had his first knee surgery and then again, in 1999. In 2000, he had two lower back surgeries. His friends thought he simply loved going under the knife when actually, Dr Joshi was extremely clear. Back then, he was a consultant to the Board of Control for Cricket in India (BCCI) and MRF Pace Foundation. Knowing what he knew about such conditions and seeing sportspeople performing at the highest level, he wanted to be physically active at any cost. He knew that surgery could, in fact, prolong his sporting lifestyle. And it indeed has.

Dr Joshi was then looking for low-impact sports. He picked scuba diving and underwater photography, but finally settled on cycling, which plays an important role in his life today. He uses it for commuting to work and it is a serious hobby. His foldable bike goes everywhere with him, even when he's travelling the country or abroad.

In 2002, Mustafa, who worked with Mercedes-Benz in Dubai, visited Dr Joshi for knee surgery. But Dr Joshi advised Mustafa against an operation. The patient was surprised to hear this from a surgeon. Dr Joshi had a simple message for him, which should be an important one for all surgeons:

'A good surgeon is one who knows when not to operate.'

Mustafa was thankful for not having been made to undergo unnecessary surgery.

If there happens to be a need for surgery and a wish to get back to any level of physical activity, whether it be for leisure, health or competition, it is important to consider a number of factors that will determine the rate of recovery and long-term health, as opined by Dr Joshi.

Dr Gurinder Bedi, head of the department and director of orthopaedics, Fortis Flt. Lt. Rajan Dhall Hospital, Delhi, has been active all his life but isn't much of a gym person. Whenever he travels for conferences around the world, he goes out for walks and runs although not for very long distances. But he loves to explore new places on his feet as much as he can. He picked up running when, earlier in 2020, Rajat had put together a 'Couch to 11-km' plan, where a daily plan would be sent to the subscriber over WhatsApp. After taking up the challenge, Dr Bedi opined:

'I regret that I didn't pick up exercising and running sooner as I am at the wrong end of 50s and now appreciate its importance.'

Dr Bedi further shared his thoughts on the role of rehabilitation in his surgical practice.

'Rehabilitation is the main thing. Frankly, you can actually make out who is going to do well or not do well based on their motivation for rehab. The worst kind of patients are those who get into surgery and think that they have done their bit and now someone else [is] going to do it for them. That is never going to work out. So the first question for me to the question is, how motivated are you. Pick your right patients up. If you have a patient who is going to get surgery done and then lie down on a couch, you might as well give up on him or her. Pick your patients right at the beginning. Tell them about the course of treatment. Tell them that, look, this is not a one-day kind of thing. This is going to take a few weeks, maybe even months. If you want to get the best out of it, your participation is as important as ours, and you need to get a professional on board, whether you get a physiotherapist, a personal trainer, or a yoga expert, it's up to your comfort zone, but if you are not even going to rehab, then don't get the surgery done. Once you introduce them to a few people who've been through it, they're

actually pretty much engaged with it right from the beginning.
The ones who aren't interested, will just drop out right there
and say that's it not for me. So I think my conversation is fairly
big with them in terms of what I want and expect from them.'

Following surgery, the primary concern must be to ensure
there is no negative impact on the immediate outcome of
the surgery by engaging in strenuous exercise too soon. You
should consult with your surgeon prior to the surgery, to make
them aware that you wish to return to exercise and sports as
soon as possible. You will then be able to discuss a suitable
plan and make sure that the surgeon is 'on board' with your
ambition. If you are working with a physiotherapist following
surgery, you must inform them about your ambitions to
return to running. This can have a large influence on the level
of function that is sought in recovery.

Surgery will cause a degree of inflammation and oxidative
stress and you will also most likely be required to rest (be it
full bed rest, or otherwise) for a period of time post-surgery.
These processes together will contribute to a degree of muscle
wasting (weakening), so minimizing the amount of rest before
returning to basic activities of daily living (walking, climbing
stairs, etc.) is essential. This will depend on the extent of
surgery but can be less than 8 weeks post operation.

As part of this process, there is a chance to return to
the very basics of movement, be it walking or running gait,
getting up from a chair, etc. Returning to the fundamentals of
movement patterns following surgery ensures that you develop
the right habits which will support long-term musculoskeletal
health. It is also important to return to the basics of resistance
exercises which will increase strength and transfer to your

running performance e.g., squats, donkey kicks, heel raises, etc. Performing these exercises in a unilateral (one leg) as well as bilateral (both legs together) fashion makes sure that you are not developing compensatory movement patterns. Asking your trainer or coach to monitor your exercises, watching in a mirror, or videoing them for yourself to review later are all good ways to ensure you are doing them right. The aim should be to restore normal function.

Nutrition is also fundamental when recovering from surgery in order to provide the necessary macro and micro nutrients required to regenerate damaged tissues. Another factor in the recovery from surgery, which is often overlooked, is your state of psychological well-being.

There is now evidence to suggest that pain 'catastrophization', i.e., the tendency to magnify the threat value of pain stimulus and to feel helpless in the context of pain, also influences the outcomes following surgery. Setting your goal of returning to exercise, running, sports and also seeking consultation and advice from a psychologist may also be suitable to aid in recovery from surgery.

9

Women's Health

Though the authors aren't women, they appreciate the fact that women are the nucleus of society. The powerhouse that's always working in stealth mode. If it wasn't for women, there would be no society, or even a human race.

It might come as a surprise to those who have forgotten the history they learnt in class nine, but in the early Vedic age, women were treated as equal to men. We are talking about 1500 to 1000 BCE, i.e., over 3000 to 3500 years ago. Then came along the later Vedic age, i.e., approximately 1000 to 500 BCE, when women were made to assume a subordinate position. Sadly, it hasn't changed much in modern society.[1]

It wasn't an anomaly. There was an overall change in society. In the early Vedic age, the king served his people and the sabha and samiti were effective checks on his authority. But they were converted to the king's court in the later Vedic age, and he became all-powerful. And as we all know, power corrupts.

When it came to religion, people only worshipped nature earlier. It might interest you that the word 'bhagwan' is possibly a mnemonic for the five elements:

1. bh: bhumi (earth)
2. ga: gagan (sky)
3. w: wayu (wind)
4. aa: agni (fire)/surya (sun)
5. n: neer (water)/indra (rain)

In the later Vedic age, people started praying to many other gods, paying less attention to the original 'bhagwan', i.e., nature. Simple religion and rituals became more complicated, and priests became too powerful, dominating the lives of citizens from birth to death. People had to bribe their way through at every step of life. Overall, whether it was the king or the priest or man, everyone wanted to dominate whoever they could.

In today's healthcare space, doctors are doing what kings and priests were doing in the later Vedic age. It's time we democratize healthcare and treat everyone in society as equals, not as a favour to anyone, but because we are. We should all have that desire and awareness to be equal. After all, this isn't the later Vedic age.

That awareness that we are equal but, at the same time, different, is crucial. An interesting example in healthcare is addressing heart (cardiovascular) diseases in women. Until very recently, and in most parts of the world, even today, the way cardiac medicine is practised is based upon whatever research is done on male patients. But then, men don't get pregnant or menstruate and don't have other conditions that are unique to women. For that reason, we both put our (Rajat and Darren) egos aside, and let female doctors enlighten us about it. We also support further research to be conducted in females, so that a greater picture can develop in the years to come. In this chapter, we will focus on women's health, highlighting the many stages of a woman's life, where in modern society, health is often compromised.

Even though, for a long time, society has assumed that girls and women are weaker than boys and men respectively, that assumption, reinforced by the society we live in, is not backed by science. The next time your sister, daughter or niece is told to act like a girl, tell them what it actually means.

* * *

Desmond Morris, a zoologist, observed in his book, *The Naked Woman: A Study of the Female Body*[2] that at the age of thirty, the average man could have 28 kg of muscle, compared to 15 kg for the average woman. This leads to the average male being 30 per cent stronger, 10 per cent heavier and 7 per cent taller. But contrary to what you would expect, this doesn't make men more robust than women.

The female body is designed for reproduction, an endurance race like no other. Women are better protected against starvation. The average woman's curvaceous body contains approximately 30 per cent fat, while a stringy male has less at approximately 20 per cent (although in the age of obesity, this can be much greater.[3] This gives women an edge over men when it comes to enduring pain and endurance sports such as distance running, where you must burn fat, and fight pain and fatigue.

In 2011, during the second edition of La Ultra, Ray Sánchez, a former American three-time Golden Glove boxer, was leading the 222-km run in Ladakh (Indian Himalayas) till about 160 km by over 4–5 hours. Sharon Gayter, a forty-

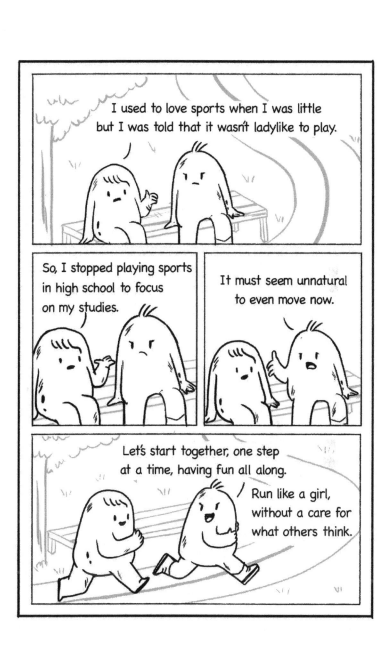

seven-year-old, was in the second spot. At that time, Ray was the only runner in the world to have completed four of the toughest 217-km ultramarathons globally (the BAD Cup 135 series, known as the world's toughest foot race) in a calendar year.

Sharon was no novice as she was Britain's top female 24-hour runner for the past 12 years, but at the end of La Ultra, she also recognized what kind of a race she had just run.

> 'I have done over 1000 races and this is 100 per cent the toughest. It is head and shoulders above the rest. The challenge of altitude is monstrous compared to heat, and this had heat and cold as well. The Badwater Ultramarathon[4] in the US, often touted as the toughest, wouldn't compare with La Ultra because heat, the main challenge at Badwater, can be handled with the runner's crew spraying water on the athlete and so on. In contrast, there is nothing one can do about high altitude leading to the lack of oxygen.'

Sharon's comments were even more important as she is asthmatic and the biggest challenge in Ladakh is the air's low oxygen content that can make the fittest struggle to do strenuous activities without appropriate acclimatization and training. Sharon observed that her regular inhaler wouldn't work at those heights because of the pressure difference, so she had to use a nebulizer every 4 hours. That was the only year that either an inhaler or nebulizer was allowed without the person being disqualified from the race.

The race had started from an altitude of about 13,500 feet, 10 km from Khardung village, where they had camped for the night, on the road to Nubra valley. For the first 42 km, a full marathon distance, the route was all uphill till Khardung La at 17,700 feet, which was claimed as the highest motorable mountain pass in the world till a road was constructed crossing Umling La at 19,204 feet.[5] Here, oxygen content can be as low as 60 per cent of what we breathe on the plains. Ray had opened up a massive gap between him and Sharon who was in the second place.

At night, the weather was bad. It was cold and reported to be snowing at the high passes. Luckily, they had crossed the passes during the day. The racecourse, around 100 km, passed through the city of Leh. Sharon found the stretch from Leh to Choglamsar the worst because of the traffic and the forever suspended exhaust smoke due to thin air.

Even though Sharon normally doesn't rest much during her races, she had to take a break as she was struggling because of exhaustion and laboured breathing. On the other hand, Ray decided to follow a different strategy. He didn't take a break to rest as he had planned to finish the race in under 30 hours. Even though it looked all good for Ray, he started hallucinating at the top of Tanglang La, the second mountain pass that needed to be crossed. He saw penguins and waves rushing towards him.

Sharon, an asthmatic who should have supposedly struggled in such conditions, not only caught up with him, but also beat Ray by an hour and a half, finishing in 37 hours and 34 minutes.

In the first ten editions of La Ultra, a total of fifty-three participants have attempted the 222-km category and only one has had a better finish time than Sharon. So much for women being the weaker sex!

About a decade earlier, in 2002, Pam Reed, a 100-pound (45 kg) parent to five children, ran the Badwater Ultramarathon that Sharon has mentioned in her experience, covering 217 km non-stop from Death Valley to Mount Whitney, California, in temperatures up to 55 degrees Celsius. She beat the course record (for either sex) by more than 5 hours.

In 2003, she again made history when she braved the hottest weather in years to successfully defend her title, defeating celebrated ultra-runner Dean Karnazes.[6]

In Constantina Diță,[7] we had another great example of what women (and mothers) are capable of. It wasn't just that she became an Olympic champion in Beijing (2008) in a field where she didn't count among the big names. Nor was it that she won after losing 4 months' training time to a leg injury in 2007. Not even that she divorced, just before the Olympics the man who was also her coach which led to a 4-month professional split as well. It was that at thirty-eight, she became the oldest woman to win the Olympics marathon by eight years.

Another ultramarathon runner, Siri Terjesen was diagnosed with scoliosis (abnormal curvature of the spine) at age seven. She wore a full body brace for nine years and was able to remove it for just an hour each day. She was left temporarily immobilized when, at sixteen, two steel rods were implanted in her back, from the top of her neck to her tail bone. Now, at 33, a professor at Indiana University, she has run about 100 marathons and ultramarathons. She won the 100-km UK championship, 50-km titles in Australia and England, and a 40-mile title in Wales. Although an American citizen, she was named British Ultra Runner of the Year in 2003. She won the 50-km 2008 Cowtown women's ultramarathon in Fort Worth, and the Cowtown marathon in 2007. Not only was she the first woman to finish at the 2008 Cowtown, but she came third overall.[8] Two places behind her was another woman, Gert Freas.

Women weren't even allowed to compete in the Boston marathon, a mere 42.195 km, until 1972. Till 1984, they were not permitted to compete in the Olympics. And here they are now.

Ladies, your bodies are awesomely well designed. Make the most of them, treat them the way they deserve to be treated. Get up, put on your shoes and prove everyone who said, 'It's not for women' wrong.

* * *

Pregnancy is one of the most natural events that a woman can go through in her lifetime. However, many women are now suffering with significant complications related to fertility, pregnancy and childbirth.

Less than 15 per cent of women end up doing the recommended 30-minute exercises, five times a day during their pregnancy. Depression is 25 per cent lesser and the risk of developing gestational diabetes, hypertension and preeclampsia is 40 per cent lower in women who are active during their pregnancy. With improvement in nutrition and reduction in obesity, infertility rates reduce.[9]

Whilst a woman is pregnant, the safety and health of the growing baby is rightly the woman's utmost concern. This concern has led to many women and their families believing that it is unsafe for a woman to undertake exercise during pregnancy.

To ensure that women and their babies are healthy before, during and after childbirth, Dr Erika Patel,[10] an obstetrician and gynaecologist, and a fertility specialist, is now working extremely hard to dispel this myth.

When she was over 6 months pregnant, Dr Patel was running three times a week. This physical credibility, alongside her strong academic and medical qualifications, has really helped her patients. Dr Patel shares her journey:[11]

'I am a doctor, a runner and a mother.

I was born and brought up in Ahmedabad. I did my MBBS and M.S. Obstetrics and Gynecology and continue to study further to finish my M.Ch in Reproductive Medicine and Surgery. I now practice in Chennai as a fertility specialist at ART fertility clinics and I am also pursuing my Phd in the same subject.

I have been an athlete all my life. I played state level badminton for Gujarat state while I was in school. However, once I shifted to Chennai, I lost touch with fitness for a few years. I started running back in 2015 with the initial intention of losing weight and getting back in shape. I remember it being a one-minute run and 3-minute walk as my first run. I also started strength training on alternate days. I joined Chennai runners in 2016 and I was guided by them on how to progress further in running longer distances. I have come a long way since then.

Running marathons is now more of a passion. I have run several short distance races 10-21 km. However, my biggest achievement was running my first full marathon in Berlin, Germany. I have a one year old baby boy and a hectic work life, but I still try to wake up early in the morning to get that run in. It is my relaxing time and gives me a lot of energy to start my day on a positive note.

I always knew that I was going to continue running throughout pregnancy. Being an ob-gyn I knew the importance of exercise in pregnancy. It wasn't the same as before, but I am glad I was able to continue till the day I delivered. I enrolled with Coach Lindsey Parry who has previously worked with a lot of pregnant athletes. All my runs were now run-walks with the aim of keeping the heart rate low. I continued my strength training with The Quad (Bootcamp workouts) where they guided me in a very trimester-based exercise routine and I also did my prenatal yoga with Dr Sonali Santhanam (a physical therapist with an interest in women's pelvic health, an evidence-based birth, childbirth educator and a certified prenatal yoga teacher). There were good days and there were bad ones. But I learned the importance of listening to my body. I ran a 10k race when I was 30 weeks pregnant. My slowest one but still the most memorable one. In my entire journey of running in pregnancy, I was very clear in my mind that if at any point I need to stop I will listen to my body and not feel dejected by it. Right then the COVID-19 pandemic hit us and all I had was a 100 metre driveway in my house to do my workouts. The restrictions that came with the lockdown was the toughest challenge I had to overcome from a mental perspective. I am very thankful to my baby for being so patient with me throughout. I constantly monitored the well being of the baby and made sure that everything was fine. In spite of being a gynaecologist I did a lot of research about exercise in pregnancy and I would like to put this out here that every woman is different and every pregnancy is different. So, my advice would be to make all the decisions after getting it cleared from your gynaecologist.

Exercise in pregnancy helps you stay active, prevents excessive weight gain, gestational diabetes and also helps in prevention of pre-eclampsia. It is safe in absence of contraindications provided you were doing it even before conceiving. It is very important to not start anything new and strenuous once you are pregnant. I realised that the biggest advantage of being active in pregnancy is actually postpartum recovery. I had a 30-hour labour and I was back on my feet that very day. Thanks to all the workouts I did while I was carrying. I slowly started my postpartum recovery in a phased manner under guidance from my coach and pelvic therapist. I ran a 21k at 21 weeks postpartum and I ran my fastest 10k, improving my personal best by over 5 minutes, at 7 months post delivery.

In my field of fertility medicine, I see so many patients with PolyCystic Ovarian Syndrome (PCOS) and obesity which leads to infertility and hence I can not stress this enough that being active is so very important at any stage of your life.'

The syndrome Dr Patel is alluding to is often characterized by infertility and causes many complications and suffering. About 25–30 years ago, PCOS was mentioned in medical textbooks but wasn't seen enough in clinics. Today, this condition is reported at epidemic levels and although the exact cause is unknown, a combination of genetic and rampant sedentary lifestyle factors are most likely factors. Dr Patel suggests that with as little as a 5 per cent reduction in body fat, it is possible for women who could not ovulate due to PCOS to begin natural ovulation.

Dr Priyanka Mantri, a dermatologist who runs and exercises, has been on a journey of fitness from a point of severe back pain. She now recommends and encourages her patients to undertake exercise as the foundation before any medical intervention. She revealed that many patients she consults have PCOS due to an imbalance in hormones. Knowing that these hormones are influenced by lifestyle factors, she questions her patients on whether they are physically active and if they eat a balanced, healthy diet. She makes inquiries about their mental well-being as well because we now know that anxiety and depression can play a role in PCOS. On the other hand, PCOS itself is associated with inflammation throughout the body, which is further associated with high cortisol levels, that can cause depression and anxiety.

It's good to know about Dr Mantri's holistic approach when most doctors are treating the symptoms of PCOS rather than causes, leading to the prescription of contraceptives and even drugs to help with the management of blood sugar. Such drugs are often prescribed with no estimation as to how long they will be needed and do not address the social and behavioural issues related to a poor lifestyle.

Dr Anjali Kumar, the renowned obstetrician, gynaecologist, laparoscopic surgeon and fertility specialist in Gurugram with rich expertise of more than 30 years, is bucking the trend in this field. A qualified yoga instructor, something she believes in as much as her medical degree, and as someone who is a physical fitness enthusiast, she is challenging long-held social and cultural beliefs around what a 'healthy' weight is by promoting exercise as the most important armour against PCOS.

* * *

Exercise and *MoveMint* need to be encouraged in early life, promoting positive behaviour that has a profound effect on physical growth and development as well as psychological, emotional and social benefits. However, encouraging girls and young women to be active and remain active is a challenge. Society often reminds girls from a young age how 'unladylike' it is to be active and sporty which is a view that can have a lasting negative impact. Many young women abandon physical activity and sport when they leave school, although certain campaigns such as the 'This Girl Can' campaign in the UK,[12] are starting to gain momentum. For those women who become increasingly sedentary, simple everyday tasks and even the act of conscious walking can begin to cause problems leading to musculoskeletal issues and other health problems.

One of the many challenges that young women have as a potential barrier to exercise is their menstrual periods. Monthly cyclical bleeding is normal for healthy women in the reproductive age group. Up to a quarter of them are affected by heavy menstrual bleeding which can also be coupled with period pains lasting up to a week and repeating every 4 weeks. That can add up to a quarter of their lifetime over three decades which happen to be their prime years. Since there is such a taboo talking about this, it becomes tricky to know what is normal or not. It is then helpful to define heavy menstrual bleeding as per Dr Kumar's definition that 'women's perception of increased menstrual volume regardless of regularity, frequency or duration', as done by the International Federation of Gynaecology and Obstetrics. Dr Kumar adds to the definition as, 'excessive menstrual blood loss which interferes with physical, social, emotional or material quality of life'.

Besides emotional and psychological strains, there are some very practical issues as well of having heavy menstrual bleeding and trying to be physically active and sporty. During periods, passing large clots, frequent need for changing sanitary napkins and staining clothes can be disturbing for even the most confident women who may have normal bleeding during periods. This affects sports performance and fitness activities in almost all women.

There is a physical impact too. Women who experience heavy bleeding are usually low on haemoglobin (anaemia) and iron, leading to fatigue, sluggishness and tiredness not only limited to their periods but throughout. This is accompanied by mood swings and anxiety. Somehow, they are not able to make the connection and get injured, as they then overdo exercises in their eagerness to cover up for the lost days of running or training in the gym.

Most women today rediscover physical exercises and running after a few decades and, at that age, having bleeding even in between periods shouldn't be ignored. If it's been there for more than 3 months, please do meet your gynaecologist. If ladies above the age of 45 years start to experience heavy menstrual bleeding or it starts getting worse, it's something to pay attention to. Dr Kumar adds that new onset of heavy menstrual bleeding, consistently heavy and prolonged periods with pain, any associated abnormal vaginal discharge, any mass or lump in the abdomen and any associated medical conditions like diabetes, need medical attention.

This also plays havoc in the lives of young, active girls at the very onset of periods when they experience painful, heavy bleeding. Some of them get into their cocoon and are never able to come out of it. There is a need for psychologists to be engaged as well as the taboo makes under-reporting the norm.

Dr Kumar adds:

'Heavy blood flow can be managed by using large sanitary pads, tampons or menstrual cups. Chafing because of continuously using a pad can be reduced by using cotton pads and by frequently changing them. Frequent chafing and wet pads can predispose a woman to fungal infections in the genital area and groin. Using an antifungal powder topically can prevent these infections. Tampons and menstrual cups are a better option in case of running during rains. Usually, there is no fear of tampon or a menstrual cup slipping away during a run if the size is correct.'

Most women have to come to terms with heavy bleeding but pain is what bothers them a lot. A large number of women report that when they run and exercise during periods, as much as they can, it helps them to have less period pain and cramps during, before and after periods. It also starts reducing their bleeding days.

Please get moving and run like a girl, becoming a role model to all around!

We also need to remember that women doctors still have their own challenges. Dr Linda George, an obstetrician and gynaecologist, shares her experience of trying to juggle between the roles of mother of two young boys and being a doctor.

'In this day and age we see women's career has taken precedence over motherhood. So we find many women between the ages of 32-37 yrs coming to us with their first pregnancy. Some of

them have an easy conception, others, assisted. We also see that due to the sedentary lifestyle, polycystic ovarian disease is on the rise which also contributes to the difficult or delayed conception. Many studies say that the ideal childbearing age is from 22-35yrs. With increasing maternal age, the risk of complications also increases. Complications like decreased fertility, Downs syndrome, increased risk of miscarriage and Caesarian deliveries, pregnancy induced hypertension, low birth weight babies, still birth or multiple births, gestational diabetes, post partum depression to name a few.

I for one got married at the age of 27 which is considered quite late down south (India). I had my first son at the age of 31 yrs following ovulation induction and Follicular Imaging. My pregnancy was a walk in the park. My mother-in-law thought I was faking my pregnancy as I didn't have any of the usual pregnancy symptoms. Following a Caesarean delivery (for cephalopelvic disproportion) on my 3rd postoperative day, when my doctor came for rounds, she was surprised to see me sitting on the floor and eating, which is a custom in Tamil Nadu. She discharged me the following day.

My second son was conceived at the age of 39, following 2 yrs of on and off fertility treatment, by intrauterine insemination (as my eldest son was praying for a sibling for 4 yrs). I developed gestational diabetes and anaemia. Post Caesarean, I developed paralytic ileus and was in so much pain that I was not able to lie flat on my back for almost 10 days.

My mother-in-law had 3 children plus a tubectomy by the age of 23. I saw how she was able to manage her household and take good care and even play with her grandchildren.

In terms of taking care of both of my boys I found that I had more energy and was in better form in my 30's compared to my 40's. Many would say that it is only normal and natural. I had gained a lot of weight (post second pregnancy) and found it very difficult to attend to my boys. That's when I decided that I needed to do something about my health. I am and never have been very athletic but for the past two years I have been walking at least 30 minutes a day followed by some spot exercises. I find it relaxing, a time to contemplate and also plan my day. As a working woman and single mother of 2 boys, the younger one being 5 years, I try not to miss exercising in the mornings as something always comes up in the form of work or family emergencies after that. 30 minutes of regular walking may not be much, but in the long run it definitely has its health benefits. For me, the major benefit is that now, after losing a few kilos (I also try to follow intermittent fasting whenever possible), I am able to keep up with my younger son, am more attentive and less cranky, have more energy to play and spend with my boys compared to before, and overall it is a great feeling.[13]

In 2004, during Aparna Ramachandra's first caesarean section, the epidural was botched up and she developed severe back pain. It would take Aparna, the managing director of RectifyCredit, more than 20 minutes to sit up to feed her baby. Over the next few months, it got even worse. Physical inactivity like never before led to weight gain. When her son was 10 months old, she decided that she had had enough and vowed to get back in shape. To start with, even, 2 km felt like a trek. Over the next 3 months, she managed to climb the top of a small steep hill, covering a distance of 7.5 km. And in 18 months, she lost 23 kg and felt fabulous.

Just when she thought she was in control, she experienced her second episode of severe back pain. This grounded her for 8 weeks. She slowly started to get back to life again, but in less than a year, she had neck and shoulder pain that was diagnosed as frozen shoulder. At times, it was extremely painful to be mobile.

However, since 2004, she managed to exercise 4–5 days a week, as much as she comfortably could. It could be going to the gym, a walk or whatever worked.

She turned forty years old in January 2015 and wanted to push her body to do physical activities that she hadn't done so far in her life but saw women around her do. She had been hearing about the Mumbai marathon for over a decade but she had never run before. She decided to go for the half-marathon there. She trained well with a running group for 4 months.

As luck would have it, three days before the race, her back gave way, reminding her of her previous episodes. But on the morning of the race, she woke up and told her body, 'Baby, you and I have to do this together.' She started the race slow and steady, with one small step at a time.

Soon she found her rhythm. On getting to the dreaded Peddar Road flyover, just 4–5 km short of the finish line, she got a bit nervous about her back. As a precautionary measure, she applied anti-inflammatory spray that was available at the nearby aid station. That was an expensive mistake, as it only added to the discomfort. Her back was on fire and went into a spasm that she hadn't experienced before. Luckily, an elderly gentleman standing nearby noticed this and kept her company for the next 1.5 km. The last 3 km were run by her mind, and not by her body.

Since then, she has run multiple half-marathons, but only with a good 3–4 months of training before each race. In 2020, she was part of the group of 26 women who were running from Pune to Mumbai, a distance of 168 km in 2.5 days. They took rest breaks at night.

She isn't a superfast runner who is representing the country and breaking any records, but she tries to be her best each day, better than she was the day before. Mentally, she is stronger than ever before.

Aparna's thoughts on her running are simple but deep.

'We need not get inactive and give up on life. We have only one life to live and I want to live it well. These setbacks have only been reminders from my body. The mind is more powerful than the body. Whether it is for losing weight, running or cycling, it is all in our mind. If we decide, then nothing can stop us.'[14]

* * *

Rajat had taken his wife, Nidhi, to Jomsom in Nepal, thinking that she would love it. She happened to be 6 months pregnant at that time. To make matters worse, even though she was petite, she wasn't adventurous and was extremely sedentary. Jomsom is at an altitude of 8900 feet in western Nepal, with very similar geography to Ladakh. It was a steep climb to the hotel and if Nidhi had her way, she would have taken the flight back right then. From then, Nidhi started to gain weight and was extremely sedentary for two decades till 2020. In 2020, she started walking for an hour a day. Then, she started to run a bit. Now, Nidhi and Rajat go out together for a run and do an hour or two a day, courtesy of which, Rajat says, that she is in a much better health and mood all the time. Running buddies end up spending a lot more quality time together than they would spend with their partners, and it's even better if they happen to be partners who exercise together. It is Nidhi who makes sure that Rajat is disciplined to go out running regularly now.

The postnatal period is a critical time, not only for the baby, but also for the recovery of the mother. If the mother does not take care of herself in the initial period after birth, there are a number of issues that can develop later. Firstly, if there is a lack of suitable nutrition, sleep and exercise (probably in that order as three key principles), then milk supply can suffer. The physiology of milk supply is vastly complex and is far beyond what we can talk about here, but needless to say, the very basics have to be in place. It is both the anatomy and physiology of the mother that dramatically changes during pregnancy and the body needs time and the right conditions to return to a healthy 'non-pregnant' state.

The muscles of the abdomen move and change shape during pregnancy to allow for the growth of the baby and also for childbirth. In fact, it is these muscles that contract and help push the baby out! The level of contraction initiated by the body is far greater than we could ever generate with basic exercises.

Darren's wife, Meena, gave birth to their second child in 2021. In order that Darren could appreciate the level of contraction that women go through in childbirth, Meena offered to take him to a facility where they place electrodes on the abdomen of men and apply electrical stimulation to simulate the contractions of childbirth. After watching some of the videos online, Darren politely declined. However, he will forever be in awe of women who bear that pain.

After childbirth, these muscles have to be 'trained' to return back to their original place and function. One thing that a lot of women can suffer from post childbirth is some degree of incontinence, where the pelvic floor muscles are too weak to support the bladder. Exercises for the pelvic floor are prescribed by most midwives and doctors, but how they are performed and how regularly they are done, massively affects the outcome. All women need the attention they deserve after childbirth to ensure they can be as healthy as they can and to be the best mothers they can.

All pregnant women (and after birth) should seek the most appropriate help for themselves. There are some fantastic medical professionals who specialize in this area, such as those who we talk about in this chapter.

Another important area to consider in women's health is menopause. It can often be a subject that is not openly talked about but is something that all women will go through at a certain stage in their life. Although it may be a difficult subject to cover, it is something that needs more attention from medical professionals and society alike. We will not go into the details of all of the common symptoms and difficulties around menopause, but rather highlight and acknowledge that we all need to be more aware of it, whether we are female or male. Menopause is caused by a critical change in many hormones as the female is ageing, which can impact physical, as well as mental health. Exercise and *MoveMint* are highly effective in counteracting many of the negative aspects of menopause. For example, in maintaining (or even increasing) bone mineral density in women who have, or are at risk of developing, osteoporosis (bone loss). As we have mentioned many times over in this book, the psychological and social benefits of *MoveMint* can also have a positive impact on life during and after menopause—it can help with mood swings, stress, anxiety and depression.

Women's health is complex, and every woman will face challenges and difficulties with their health at some point throughout life. As men, we may not be best placed to provide all the answers to improving women's health, but we hope that through the stories and content we have shared, whether you are a woman or man, you will have learnt a little on how women's health can be supported.

In the words of Maya Angelou, American poet and civil rights activist, 'when women take care of their health, they become their best friend'.[15]

10

Ageing Well

The basic cause of ageing is very straightforward: we age because our cells age, and our cells age because our telomeres get short.

—Dr William 'Bill' Andrews[1]

It was 2010. Rajat had only three participants for the inaugural edition of La Ultra, his race in Ladakh. The distance was 222 km in the extreme Ladakh conditions where oxygen content of air, at times, is as low as 60 per cent that of the plains. Temperatures varied from minus 10 degrees Celsius to 40 degrees Celsius. Everyone had predicted that it was an impossible project. And there he was, in a taxi with one of the participants, Dr William 'Bill' Andrews, who at the time was fifty-nine years of age.

In an attempt to get to know Bill, Rajat asked him what he did. Bill said, 'I want to cure ageing or die trying.' Little did Rajat know that Bill was dead serious and was an authority in the field of unlocking the molecular mechanisms of ageing, and president and CEO of Sierra Sciences in the US, a company devoted to finding ways to lengthen telomeres, thus extending human lifespan and health span.

That year, Bill ended up pulling out of the race because of medical conditions but he came back at the age of sixty-one in 2012, to finish this unfinished business in style. Most people retire from their professional lives and pretty much from life too before that age. During the 2010 race, Bill committed to Molly Sheridan, another participant, on top of Khardung La. They got married a couple of years later.

Bill happens to have an identical twin, Herrick 'Rick' Andrews. They've actually got DNA sequencing done to make sure that they are 100 per cent identical twins. But Bill points out that 'identical just doesn't come from genes, it also comes from environment and lifestyle'.[2]

There is a good reason that Bill points this out. Up until the age of fifty, no one could make out who was who. They did look identical. But Bill has been a runner throughout and Rick hasn't. Bill has been mindful of his diet but Rick loves his big hamburgers, French fries and beers. Bill, on the other hand, is vegan and does not use oil for cooking. He doesn't drink alcohol. His last drink was about eighteen years ago.

At the biological age of sixty-six, they got tested for their telomere length. Bill's telomere length was that of someone forty-one and a half, whereas Rick's was that of seventy. Rick didn't seem too old for his actual age, but now, when they would stand next to each other, they did look very different. If not for their identical smile, it was difficult to even make out that they were brothers, leave alone identical twins.

At the age of sixty-nine, Rick suffered a stroke, after less than 3 months of his second bypass surgery. As for Bill, he runs a minimum of 3.2 km a day. He hasn't missed a day in over 500 days now. His present streak started in May of 2020. He has also been competing in virtual and COVID-safe marathons, 10-km races, etc. But he hasn't done an ultramarathon since the pandemic started. He can run marathons with all the water and food he needs in his camelback. But, for longer races, he would need to refill at aid stations, and he is of the opinion that wouldn't be COVID-safe enough for him. Every run is a new adventure, normally on trails. He also works out in his own private COVID-safe gym three times a week. He hasn't missed a workout in over 3 months.

When Rajat reached out to Bill in 2020, it felt like déjà vu from a decade ago. This is what Bill had to say about ageing and how to approach it:

'Chromosomes are shoelace like structures, and are there within each of the cells in the human body. The genes that give us our hair colour, our eye colour etc are 109 organized along these shoe laces. Think of these shoelaces as a computer ribbon that has data along, that's where our DNA is.

And as the tips of our shoelaces have caps called egglets to protect the ends of the shoelaces from opening up, so do our chromosomes have telomeres at the ends. These fine thread-like telomeres get shorter each time our cells divide. The basic unit of telomeres is nucleotides. When we are first conceived, the telomeres in our single-cell embryos are approximately 15,000 nucleotides long. Our cells divide rapidly in the womb, and by the time we are born, our telomeres have decreased in length to approximately 10,000 nucleotides. They shorten throughout our lifetime, and when they reach an average of about 5,000 nucleotides, our cells cannot divide any further, and we die of old age. Effectively, telomeres are a 'biological clock of aging'.

Simple cell division is a normal process that is going on all the time in our body. Some parts of our body have cell division all the time including our immune system, gut and skin, so we have a fixed rate of telomere shortening. Also there is a basal rate of telomere shortening that we can't get below. If we had the perfect genetics and led a perfect lifestyle, and didn't get run over by any bus or get into any accident, we would actually live to be 125. The rate of telomere shortening and those cells that divide all the time, limit our lifespan so that we cannot live beyond 125 years. So nobody in documented recorded history has ever lived to be a 125. Since nobody lives a perfect lifestyle, we end up living shorter.

Telomeres also shorten faster when we lead an unhealthy lifestyle including increased stress, poor quality sleep, smoking, sedentary life etc. That is called accelerated aging.

So, one of the best things that you can do to slow down shortening of your telomeres is endurance exercise. But it has a goldilocks effect. If you rarely do any exercise, then that's going to cause accelerated telomeres shortening because your body is going to be in an inflamed state. Just getting up out of the chair to climb up the stairs or something like that, is going to cause inflammation. So the trick is to be active regularly, not occasionally and definitely not be a slob forever. And enjoy the run, have fun, that's the best way to approach running or exercise.'[3]

Rather than blaming your parents, it's entirely up to you how you express your genes. And now is a good time to get started. Bill admits that till the age of fifty, he too loved foods like French fries but then he changed his diet. And today, at seventy, he told Rajat that he wants to run 666 km at La Ultra.

Even though Darren is only thirty-four years old (at the time of writing), some days, when he gets up early in the morning, or after a long day, he feels 'old'. However, the one thing that makes him feel younger is when he gets moving! When people get beyond their twenties, they are often told, why carry on playing any sport if they no longer are planning to go to the Olympics. Rajat was definitely told that at the age of eighteen when he had retinal detachment and needed surgery. At that time, he was into long-distance running and weight training. The fascinating part is that he's run far longer and done far more strength training after the retinal detachment way back in 1993.

From the moment we are born, we are ageing. When a child is just a few minutes old, leave alone hours, days or months, we say that they are 'so and so' many minutes old. Ageing is looked at differently in different cultures; a non-starter when it comes to being physically active. Too often, patients are told not to be active any more because they have reached thirty years of age, forget any further. In India, till about a decade ago, and even now, in most families, it is considered that once someone has retired from work, i.e., reached their late fifties or early sixties, depending on the nature of work or department, it is time to not only retire from work but from life itself. Ageing is a fact of life and something that affects us all. That is why we wanted to include it in this book as a main chapter. If followed carefully, the advice that is given could have the greatest impact on your life and others you love too.

Physiologically, there are changes in the human body. Bone density reduces and muscle loss happens. But what is fascinating, as mentioned on the *MoveMint Medicine* podcast by Dr Bradley Elliot, an exercise physiologist who researches the effects of exercise on ageing, is that all that can be markedly slowed and even reversed with exercise and *MoveMint*. Age is literally a number and at any age, there is no reason to stop exercising. On the contrary, there is more of a reason to exercise as you age.

Seventy-seven-year-old Surgeon Captain Dr Jagbir Singh Nagra (retired) is, today, a lot more active than he has ever been. He admits that only when he retired at the age of seventy—you read that right—that too reluctantly, by his standards, did he focus on physical activities. Prior to that, there was more focus on work, but he did walk extensively even then. He now devotes 2.5 hours to walking, running and exercising, paying him good dividends. Dr Nagra pointed out that medical college was hectic and as a doctor in the army and navy, one could miss out on drills and sports. He has signed up for running his first run, 11 km at La Ultra in 2022, and would have most probably run by the time you read this. It was in 2004, a ninety-five-year-old, rather 'young' gentleman walked into Rajat's clinic in London. He told him that he had no pain and wanted to pick up strength training to get even fitter. Fauja Singh (sadly no longer alive) was a farmer in India but had only picked up running at the age of eighty-four after moving to the UK. That same year, as a ninety-three-year-old, he was featured on Adidas' advertisement campaigns all across London. The hoardings bragged about his finish times for full marathon (42 km): '6 hrs 54 minutes at age 89; 5 hrs 40 minutes at age 92. The Kenyans had better watch out for him when he hits 100.' So, what actually happens in ageing and how do people like Dr Nagra and Singh manage to stay so active and healthy in old age?

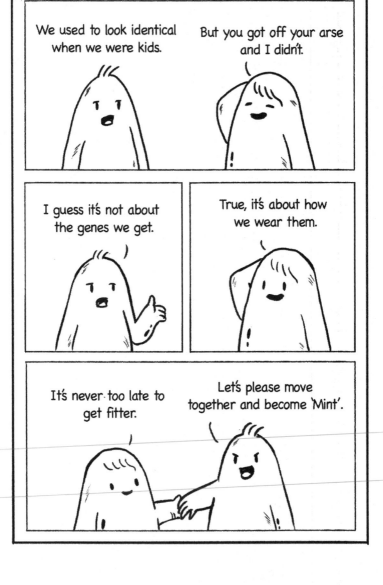

With ageing, your muscles get weaker, your bones get a little bit less dense and they can break a little easier. We all have family members or friends who have become frailer as they age, a phenomenon that often creeps up on people very quickly from their sixth decade of life. Although we may not become frail until later in life, many of the mechanisms that contribute to ageing begin to deteriorate surprisingly early on. For example, we can lose as much as 1 per cent of our total muscle mass per year, from the age of forty. This might not seem like a lot, but as the years pass by, this can have a huge impact on our ability to undertake the most basic daily tasks. This just means you need to start being active if you haven't already been. And if you already have been active, become even more active.

In fact, we now know that in ageing, muscle mass can contribute to morbidity and mortality. Frailty isn't just something that we see in the elderly and accept; it is a clinical condition which can be diagnosed and, in many cases, managed. Muscle wasting in ageing is known as 'sarcopenia' which is derived from the Latin, 'poverty of flesh'.

This implies that the person is in a place of great need. But in ancient Greek mythology, Geras (the god of old age) was revered as a figure of fame, excellence and courage. This was despite Geras being depicted as a tiny, shrivelled old man, often in the presence of the hero, Heracles, the son of Zeus and Alcmene. In fact, the related word, 'géras' was used in ancient Greek literature to carry the meaning of influence, authority and power. In modern society, many of us look to our elders for advice and wisdom in the challenges that we face, something that has not changed in thousands of years.

However, the biggest challenge that we face in the world today, is a rapidly expanding population with an ever-increasing life expectancy, courtesy advancements in the healthcare industry. It doesn't help living longer if the quality of life is majorly compromised. What we need to be pushing towards is a place of healthy ageing, where we can all live healthy, independent lives through to old age and death.

So how are we going to do this? Exercise and *MoveMint*, along with good mental health, sleep and eating habits have to be at the centre of this goal. As we have briefly mentioned above, exercise can really counteract a lot of physiological changes that we see in ageing. There is a lot of evidence now to indicate that resistance exercise leads to gains in muscle strength and bone density. The term 'resistance exercise' is relative to the individual. So, for an elderly individual even resisting against something very light in weight, e.g., a water bottle, can be sufficient to begin to improve strength. It doesn't have to be push-ups or lifting weights in the gym. Most people think that once they have reached a certain age, they are 'too old' to start with any form of exercise. This just cannot be the case, as has been seen by Rajat in his clinic and the many millions on TV who have witnessed Singh running alongside former professional footballer David Beckham.

In essence, the most important factor, with any exercise of *MoveMint*, is the element of progressive overload. You have to be doing more and more over time to continue to see improvements, which will be seen very quickly if you are starting from scratch.

* * *

As we age, there is an increasing chance that we will suffer from so-called age-related diseases. Whether it is musculoskeletal disease (e.g., osteoarthritis), cardiovascular disease (e.g., heart issues, high blood pressure, etc.), metabolic disease (e.g., diabetes) or neurological disease (e.g., Alzheimer's), resistance and aerobic/endurance exercise can not only help to prevent such diseases, but also help in management and treatment. There are many studies which show that those people who have continued to exercise as they age (so-called masters' athletes), have strikingly been able to stave away many diseases and conditions associated with ageing. This does not happen forever as ageing is inevitable and will catch up with us all, but we can all try to chase it away for as long as possible.

So, if you have been inactive all of your life, where is the best place to begin? Dr Elliot is immersed in the science and medicine behind this. But he recognizes the importance of psychology in promoting exercise and *MoveMint* and is working closely with psychologists to understand what is required for behavioural change to make permanent changes to our sedentary lifestyles.

Dr Elliot is of the opinion that as humans, we self-impose barriers which prevent us from starting or continuing to exercise. Throughout life, we all develop habits and our lifestyles become increasingly more restricted. Ultimately, we are often uncomfortable making changes in our lives. This becomes even more of an issue in the elderly as they will have lived their lives in a particular way for decades. So, making changes in old age can be even harder. This is why the motivation exercise and the support that is put in place needs to be thoroughly considered. This is why we advocate the *MoveMint* approach which is all about doing meaningful exercise that is fun and sustainable. It simply can't be a task as a punishment for being a naughty person.

Exercises also need to be practical and relevant to the needs of the individual. Exercises and movement that support activities of daily living are the most important in the elderly. When someone becomes frail, they often find it very difficult to get up from a chair, get up and down from the toilet, and struggle climbing stairs. Exercises can be based around targeting muscles to support these movements, with the aim of promoting independence for as long as possible.

The WHO has produced international physical activity guidelines[4] for adults aged sixty-five and above, which provide a foundation and starting point for what all adults over the age of sixty-five should be aspiring to.

More importantly, exercise and physical activity is considered in the broader sense, including leisure time activities. Such activities and hobbies are often taken up in retirement and form an essential part of continuing to engage with society. Leisure activities including walking, swimming, dancing and gardening are all promoted as forms of physical activity. Walking or cycling as modes of transport are also encouraged to further reduce the sedentary time associated with travelling by car. Although many people get assistance with household chores, cleaning the home can also be seen as a physical activity.

Taking up recreational sports in retirement is also a common thing to do. Some people are inclined to take up what might be considered more 'leisurely' sports such as golf. However, any sport or physical activity needs appropriate 'training' and thus, the foundations of *MoveMint* and exercise need to be in place. This will go some way in preventing injuries which will be more likely in old age as the musculoskeletal tissues begin to degenerate.

The main goal of physical activity in the over sixty-five age group is to improve cardiovascular health and fitness, offset the decline in musculoskeletal health, reduce the risk of non-communicable diseases (which are often age-related) and prevent depression and cognitive decline.

Older adults should at least target walks, jogs, cycling, swimming or other aerobic physical activities for 20–30 minutes daily at an intensity where their breathing increases to a level that they can only converse in sentences with seven to ten words. These guidelines are there to help you approximate intensity of the activity. Each time you do aerobics, it should be done in two to four bouts of at least 10 minutes. Of course, for additional health benefits, they can look at doing the above for an hour or even two a day.

Older adults, with poor mobility, should perform physical activity to enhance balance and prevent falls on three or more days per week. When it comes to muscle strengthening activities, focus on squats, heel raises, push-ups, etc., and do it two or more days a week.

Remember that the benefits of exercising are a lot more than physical health. It helps one unwind and relax, besides things discussed so far in the book. For most people who have been following the same routine for decades, e.g., an hour-long walk every day at the same pace, it might not be helping them immensely physically but psychologically, it is what they need. For even greater physical benefits, change the routine and push yourself a bit every few weeks the way you did when you were in school. If you were to be in class one practising single digit additions for 10 years, you would have become amazingly good at additions of single digits, but that's about it. By moving to subsequent classes every year, you improve in addition of bigger numbers and even in more complex problems like multiplication, division, etc.

These recommendations are aspirational and something that everyone should be working towards. If you are starting out, or currently seem a long way from these recommendations, do not panic. Remember, there is a positive dose response relationship with *MoveMint*, so anything is better than nothing, but more is better still. If you are suffering from a particular health condition, you should do as much physical activity as possible within your own personal limits. As you exercise more, you will come to know your body more, and hence, your boundaries and limits.

As we have discussed, there is also an increased risk of falls with ageing, which is caused by a number of factors. Balance and sensitivity of movement are compromised when we age, including central (the audio-vestibular system—inner ear) and peripheral (sensors in the muscles and joints) mechanisms. Let us simplify this further.

* * *

Dr Kshitij Malik is an audio-vestibular doctor from Gurugram, specializing in vertigo and hearing. He has some great insights into balance and its relationship with ageing and disease. To best understand the body and its myriad functions, it can be explained through the use of an analogy. Imagine a great and wise king who is the ruler of the country. He makes the most efficient judgements and takes the most prudent of actions. Since his judgements need to be based on facts, he employs an array of fact collectors. Likewise, once he carries out a judgement, he needs an army to execute them. The judgements can only be as good as the fact collector and the execution only as good as the executors of this judgement. In the case of our body's balance system, there are three fact collectors, not one. One of them is vision that gives inputs about our external environment such as 'is the floor slippery', 'is a projectile coming your way that you need to duck from' and so on.

The second fact collector is the muscle-joint sense which senses the body's orientation. This would include telling the brain if the ground where one is walking is uphill or downhill based on how much is the ankle's angle when it hits the floor; or perhaps how much is the bend of the spine when one is picking up something off the ground so that the brain knows if the centre of gravity is within the range of motion.

The third fact collector is a group of accelerometers and gyroscopes embedded in tiny bones in the deepest part of the ear that we call the vestibular labyrinth. These fact collectors can code information about how fast we are moving forward, or turning to a side, or moving up or down. Not only do they inform the brain, but as a reflex, they also make sure the image stabilizes our vision. If one is recording a video through a camera that is not still but moving all the time, the resulting video would be very shaky and poor.

If there was a way that a sensor in the camera could rapidly correct this by making the lens move in the opposite direction of the camera's movement, the resulting image would be very stable. Try focusing on any word in the passage and try to nod your head fast as if saying 'no'. If you can continue to focus on the word despite moving your head very fast, the gyroscopes and accelerometers in your head are working fine. Not only do they sense the head motion but they also give directions to the muscles around your eyes to make sure that the eyes autocorrect with respect to the head and continue to look at what they were, despite the head going hither and thither. The three points given above are the king's fact collectors, and if this was a book that liked to throw jargon at you, they can be called vision, proprioception and the vestibular system. But since it's not, we will stick with eyes, muscle-joints and the ears.

What of the king's judgement enforcers? Once the wise old king has been told about the challenges faced by the body with respect to its balance, the brain would need to tell some muscle groups to become more active and some to relax in order to maintain decent balance. For instance, if one accidentally slips on a banana peel, the eyes will notice the world slipping, the joints will tell the brain that one foot has moonwalked ahead, and the ears will sense gravity pulling the body down without inhibition. This triad is popularly termed as falling.

At this time, the brain will need to immediately execute the core muscles to pull the body to the front and use the other leg to stabilize oneself. Whether there will be a fall or not is directly related to how compliant the various muscle groups are to the brain's commands. If there have been regular drills and training sessions during happier times, the army would carry out its responsibilities with greater efficacy and prevent a fall. If not, then a fall might be inevitable.

Over his career spanning fifteen years as an audio-vestibular physician, Dr Malik has had the opportunity to analyse thousands of people who complain of concerns with their balance. One thing that has come to light is that as one ages, there is an age-associated decline in the efficiency of one's fact collectors. In Greek, as also in medical jargon, the prefix 'presby' means old. Age-associated weakness adopts the term presby, such as presbyopia (vision difficulties because of old age), presbycusis (hearing loss due to old age) and presbyvestibulopathy (balance disorder of old age). Apart from ageing, there are myriad factors that may affect people's balance. There could be disorders of the inner ear, which is primarily Dr Malik's area of interest, along with factors related to muscle-joint sense, vision or balance coordinators in the brain. This is often very distressing because movement is paramount to having a full human experience.

The helplessness of not being able to move about may cause immense psychological upheaval and despondency, and, in such situations, the sooner the healthcare providers can get the individual on their feet, the better. Dr Malik shares the case of a very pleasant seventy-year-young woman, who was fairly healthy in her day-to-day life. She had a small issue due to osteoarthritis of both knees, but not something that compelled her to make lifestyle modifications. Unfortunately, she developed an inner ear malfunction, where one of her balance organs failed all of a sudden because of a viral infection. In medical jargon, we call this vestibular neuritis. Initially, this remained undiagnosed and she ended up undergoing a series of tests and investigations, MRIs, CT scans and the works. In the end, she was told the good news that she hadn't had a stroke. Good news indeed, but it doesn't help to sort out the problem.

She met Dr Malik after 3 months of illness, during which time she was primarily on rest, which is standard medical advice that doctors give in the hope that rest gives the body the opportunity to sort out whatever the patient is suffering from. What most forget is that time itself isn't a great healer. It has the potential to heal only if we do something during that time.

During the consultation meeting, Dr Malik realized that her balance system had more or less sorted itself out when the head was stationary, but during rapid neck movements, the unsteadiness was significant. This could have been worked upon, but the disuse of major muscle groups over the last 3 months had made sure that there was little coordination and strength left in the big muscles of the legs to support her if there was even slight imbalance, and the probability of her taking a fall had become high.

Not only did she need correction for ear-related unsteadiness, but even the other balance sensor and balance executor had been compromised because of the extended period of rest. This is in contrast with another gentleman, a thirty-year-old young man who was reasonably athletic. But one day, out of the blue, he developed a similar problem, which was one-sided inner ear destruction affecting balance and hearing. Since hearing was also involved, his diagnosis was made quicker than the national average, and soon enough, he was recommended exercises and sports. While the inner ear function seldom comes back, because of early intervention, the brain adapts itself to start listening to the other fact collectors to help with balance function and decreases its reliability on the ear. Overall, balance function is retained well with no significant limitations in day-to-day activities.

Generally, when we focus on the musculoskeletal system, we tend to look at its lead role which is locomotion. However, what we often miss is that the system plays multiple roles beyond the most obvious one. It's not only the lead cast, but also the supporting cast for various other departments. Having a fit musculoskeletal system is a big help for those who might inadvertently develop inner ear diseases which may result in problems of balance. Those who have a habit of pursuing fitness tend to come out of the nasty effects of imbalance and vertigo much better and faster than their counterparts.

Due to this frailty of the musculoskeletal system, there is a vastly increased risk of serious fracture due to falls in the aged. This is particularly a problem in woman suffering from osteoporosis, where the strength of their bones is compromised, and who, courtesy the society, become inactive a lot sooner.

By far the biggest risk with falls in the elderly is the increased chance of hip fractures. These fractures can present a number of complexities and may require complex surgery to fix damaged bone structures. Surgery itself in the elderly poses significant risks with enhanced considerations for managing cardiovascular risks. Rehabilitation from surgery in the elderly is also extremely important as any degree of 'bed rest' or inactivity can exacerbate muscle wasting and weakness. Complications and other issues (also known as comorbidities) are also of serious concern with hip fracture. There are some shocking statistics related to mortality risk following hip fracture, whereby studies have reported death rates as high as 58 per cent within one year of the incident. This means that we need to prevent frailty as much as possible, by ensuring we are staying as active as far as possible as we age.

Exercise supports healthy weight maintenance and also keeps our muscles strong. This is another reason why it is thought that those who exercise have 'healthier' and 'younger' looking skin, as the skin is supported by muscle that is toned.

Whether it is the cardiovascular system, the musculoskeletal system, the brain, or the skin, exercise can prevent the process of ageing.

The most important thing is that it is a clock that never stops (until we die at least), so it is possible to have a positive impact wherever we are in our lives. This in essence is what we see in the so-called masters' athletes, where their biological age is far younger than their chronological age. Some studies have indicated that it is related to the function of the immune system which has far more roles in our body than just fighting off infection. The cells of the immune system also help with the regeneration of our tissues and are heavily involved in how our body responds to *MoveMint*.

There are a lot of misconceptions about exercising in old age, some of which have already been covered. Most people think that there is an increased risk of injury or cardiovascular events such as heart attack or stroke. However, according to a study[5] published in the *European Heart Journal*, exercise reduces the risk of heart disease and stroke in the elderly. In contrast, the authors of this study also found that decreasing physical activity as you age increases risk of cardiovascular disease. So, even if someone has been physically active throughout their life, it is still important for them to remain active in old age.

Then there are myths reinforced by our sedentary doctor colleagues that knee arthritis is caused or made worse by exercising and running later on in life.[6] That has yet again been disproved by a lot of high-quality studies. But then again, after all this evidence and experience, we keep hearing from some well-meaning doctors that 'there is an age for doing everything'. True. We guess they are the ones who don't know what all can be done.

Christine Pemberton had been active throughout her life, doing trekking and long walks, but hadn't run. She picked up running at the age of sixty. Today, at sixty-seven, she has run multiple full marathons and numerous half-marathons.

'I never thought I could run. I knew I could walk, but never thought I could run. And it has been utterly fabulous. And I am never going to stop. In my 50s I twice had knee arthroscopy for both knees. Then I was told by my surgeon that next I'll need total knee replacements. That's when I had the good fortune to meet Dr. Chauhan. On my bucket list when I turned 60 was learning how to run. Of course I had run as a child, but I had never run competitively. I had never participated in races, I had never worn a bib or crossed the finish line. And here I was at the age [of] 60 that I joined the Couch to 6k program under Dr. Chauhan's guidance, I learnt how to run. And 7 years later, I am a full marathoner. I am a slow marathoner but a marathoner. I have done eight full marathons and lots of half-marathons.'

As luck would have it, in November 2019, Christine got injured. But it had nothing to do with her running, at least not directly.[7]

'I tore the meniscus ligament in my left knee, chasing after a bunch of schoolboys who were harassing me while I was

running. I had gone for a mid-morning run in my beloved Biodiversity Park, preparing for a half marathon in December, the Mumbai Marathon in January, followed by the New Delhi Marathon in February. To my dismay I saw a huge crowd of boys – all in school uniform – on the track ahead of me. Dismay because they were shouting, and playing music and chucking chip packets on the trail – all this in a Biodiversity Park. But worse was to come.

When they saw me, despite my age, they started jeering and whistling and catcalling and filming me. Obviously I didn't back off, but sprinted past them, till I found the lone teacher – it was a huge crowd of boys, all aged about 16-18 years I'd say, taller than me, and with just one teacher. Madness. I complained about their behaviour, to which he made them all say "Sorry Madam".

Big bloody deal. Realistically, I wasn't scared that I might get attacked, but what appalled me was their pack mentality. Their brazenness. Their down right rudeness and misogyny. If they behaved like that to me, old enough to be their grandmother AND a foreigner (sometimes we get a little extra respect, but not always), then imagine had I been a young girl out alone... it actually doesn't bear thinking about.

And at some point in this awful, awful hullabaloo, I twisted my knee as I ran through the jeering crowd to find the teacher (I think I remember slipping on a stone) and bingo! Meniscus torn.

I was whimpering in agony. It hurt so much, and had to be collected from the park.

It's not the direct fault of those revolting schoolboys that I tore my meniscus. Could just as well have done it when I was running anywhere, but I didn't. I tore it while trying to deal with harassment and so those uncouth young men are part of the story.

I'll spare you the tears and the misery and the downright pain of those first few weeks.

Cancelling all my races. Hardly able to move. Weeping when my GP told me "your running days are over".

Weeping when the wonderful Dr. Chauhan subsequently told me "Rubbish, you'll run again. Ignore him!"

I had X-rays. I had an MRI. I did extensive physio. I saw an orthopaedic surgeon. Didn't run for months. Started gym. Had injections in my knees. And I can say, today, on the first anniversary of that wretched day, I am 97%-98% OK. Occasional twinges, but I'm basically OK. There is NOTHING good to be said about this injury – it cost me 3 races, dammit – BUT… If I had to be sidelined, I guess 2020 was the right year to choose, when so much has been cancelled and we've all had to spend lots of time locked down.

I can't honestly say that my injury or the enforced not-racing for a year has made me reflect on the meaning of life, or anything remotely philosophical.

What it has done, however, is make me realise that running is not simply a question of running.

Running is a w-a-y more interconnected activity than I'd initially thought, and the journey towards recovery and fitness, involving stretching and yoga and weight lifting (yes!!) has been something of an eye-opener.

It's a journey I'm actively enjoying, especially weight lifting, my latest passion.

No matter what your age is, what your physical condition is, you can stay physically active. You can start exercising. You owe it to yourself, to your family, your friends and your loved ones.'

Running and exercising gave Christine the courage to stand up against those rowdy schoolboys and also bounce back from injury to get back to running at sixty-seven.

The main focus of this chapter has been on improving quality of life and maintaining your identity as you age, but exercise and *MoveMint* can also contribute towards an increased life expectancy. As part of the Harvard alumni study,[8] researchers found that men who exercise regularly can add 2 hours to their life for every hour of exercise. Now that is not a bad investment at all! If you could get that return on financial investments (especially those that are not affected by recession), people would be spending all day and night exercising. This, in essence, is what we are advocating with *MoveMint*—exercise should be an investment that you want to make.

Whether one believes in God or not, most people do fear death. Knowing that *MoveMint* can support a better, independent, reduced disease-burdened later life, as well as potentially increasing our life expectancy, we should all be encouraged and motivated to exercise as we age.

Conclusion

I didn't have time to write you a short letter, so I wrote you a long one.

—Mark Twain

Even after having deleted more than half the stuff we wanted to say here, it's still become quite a bit. We appreciate that by now, you wouldn't remember most of what we mentioned. We most definitely don't, so we have put together some things we'll want you to get started with on your journey to an optimal happy life and get others on to it too.

Some would wonder why we didn't touch on a lot of diseases, but we weren't trying to. There are things that we would have missed, but this book is not meant to be an encyclopedia. Also, we didn't talk much about various terms like yoga and Pilates because we want you to think in a broader way and not limit yoga to just some asanas alone. Come to think of it, we spoke about yoga throughout the book without mentioning the word. After all, yoga is a way of life.

Love Yourself, Be Your Best Friend

When we hear the sentence, 'I love you unconditionally', we both just burst out laughing because love is unconditional, always should be. Else, it's a contract. So, no matter what, love yourself (unconditionally). If you don't, how do you expect anyone else to do the same for you? Be your best friend. Prioritize yourself over all others, only then can you be of any use to those whom you love with your life. For that, you need to take care of your overall health. And then you'll have a trickle-down effect.

In the words of Justin Bieber:

'Cause if you like the way you look that much
Oh, baby, you should go and love yourself.'[1]

We should love ourselves, value our life for what it is and make the most of it whilst we can.

'ProActive'

Having the thought of loving yourself unconditionally is a good start, but the thought needs to follow up with action. Rather than outsourcing your problems and looking for solutions from others, you need to be in charge and get on with being the solution yourself. Listen to all the experts out there but do what makes sense to you. After all, you are the one who has lived with yourself from the time you are born. That person across the table might have all the experience and knowledge in the world but has only known you for a few minutes. They simply can't pass a judgement, or at least, we shouldn't let them. More often than not, we are told to stop being active for good. If it's for a short while, maybe, but definitely not long term. Literally, get moving.

Smile

That movement starts with you smiling from ear to ear, for years and years. Smile, even if it's not coming from within. When others see you smiling, you'll be surprised at the number of people who will genuinely smile back, making you smile from within too. When you begin exercising, let smiling be the first step. While going out for a walk or a run, while wearing shoes, while taking a shower, just smile. Smile for no rhyme or reason. When your exercise or run gets a little hard, or you feel like stopping, just smile. You will realize that by smiling, you will be able to continue for a lot longer. Go on, smile. Now.

Don't Act Dead When Still Alive

We want you to get back to being happy, loving yourself and doing all things that you should whether you are in top health or not. There is no point dreading what'll eventually happen because no matter what, it eventually will. So why act dead before we are dead? Let's live while we are alive. Most say that 'they are dying'. It needs to change to 'they are living'. That mind shift will change how we approach life for ourselves and for all around us.

Sleep

Sleep is extremely underrated. If you exercise well and are mindful of what you eat but ignore sleep, you are doing it totally wrong. To think of it simply, what's the point of anything, if you don't sleep well at night?

Target sleeping for 7–9 hours; make an effort to sleep by 10 p.m., get done with your dinner at least 2 hours before your planned sleep time, and don't use your gadgets for an hour before while you dim the lights in your bedroom. And if you can, don't have the television in the bedroom.

Mind

Unfortunately, we all take the mind for granted, including most healthcare professionals. It's important to talk, to open up to friends, and seek professional help if need be. Psychologists and counsellors play an important role, but at the end of the day, the onus lies on you to focus on your own mental health. You need to proactively work on improving it. No one else can fix it for you while you play a passive role.

The one thing that has really worked for us is learning to let go, and the second is to appreciate that nothing is permanent.

Journey, Not the Destination

It's never a destination, always a journey. So be at it. There will be good days but don't get super excited about them. Then there will be bad days but don't get disheartened. Think of it like a long-term investment where spikes shouldn't bother us much.

Eat

Rather than jumping on to any fad diet, think for yourself, think about what'll be sustainable in your surroundings and culture. It's easy for a westerner to talk about benefits of a non-vegetarian diet, but that doesn't work in the Indian context.

We want you to focus on the basics. No matter if you are overweight or not, or even diabetic, cut down on sugar. It simply isn't good for you. While you are at it, reduce your carbohydrate intake too.

Besides everything else, fat in the food has got a bad name because of undesirable body fat. Fat is good for you. Please have ghee and dried fruits. Increase their intake.

As for proteins, they are the building blocks for your muscles. Please increase their intake. Definitely take some within 30 minutes of an exercise workout as they are important for muscle recovery and adaptation after exercises.

When it comes to hydration, most people fall in the extreme category. They either drink too much or too little. If you drink to quench your thirst, you simply won't go wrong.

Move

You may not do these things in this order, but they are things that you should do every day. Sleeping and eating are the easy things to do but being mindful and moving is sometimes more of a struggle. We moved to be born, so don't let anyone tell you otherwise. Always remember that more than exercise, it's about having an overall active lifestyle. Here are some basic movements that you can easily integrate into your life every day, which will have quick and dramatic effects on how you feel.

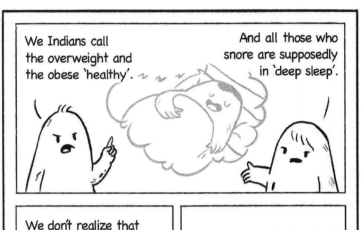

We Indians call the overweight and the obese 'healthy'.

And all those who snore are supposedly in 'deep sleep'.

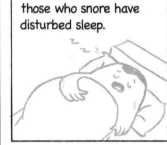

We don't realize that those who snore have disturbed sleep.

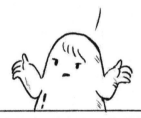

And eat a lot of junk, day in, day out.

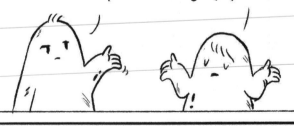

Then, every four years, the whole nation becomes an expert on winning Olympic medals.

Squats

Before we all had access to chairs, we squatted to sit, so squatting isn't an exercise but a basic instinct of being human.

Heel Raises

You do not even need to do these standing if you can't. Just raising your heels as you sit (on to your toes), will help circulate the blood from your legs back to your heart.

Orange Squeeze

This is an exercise that we should be doing multiple times a day, to avoid the poor posture that we develop from looking at our 'stupid' (also known as smart) devices. This is an exercise that will miraculously help with your breathing. Imagine that you have an orange between your shoulder blades with your elbows at 90 degrees and your fingers pointing up to the ceiling (or sky). Move your shoulders back, trying to squeeze all of the juice out of the orange. Hold the position for a few seconds and then relax. Repeat 5–10 times, depending on how you feel.

Breathing

Breathing is something that we all take for granted. Take some time throughout the day to concentrate on your breathing, being mindful of breaths in and out.

Feel

A lot of people do not take the time to feel. This could be psychological feeling (assessing how you feel), or physical feeling (taking time to appreciate the complex world around us and how we interact with it). Make sure you take some time every day to 'feel'.

Think

Similar to 'feeling', we do not take enough time to think. In our busy lives, there is often not even a second to slow down and think about anything. But in other aspects, we might 'overthink' things. So, there has to be a balance. Thinking helps us plan, evaluate and reflect, which all contribute to well-being.

Connect the Dots

Through this book, we wanted to make you think and give you some tools. But you need to think how and when they will come in handy. Fighting metabolic diseases, cancers of all kinds, infections like COVID and all other diseases are crucial, and we need to have the same approach as discussed in the book. Connect the dots and it'll all make sense.

The biggest disease the world suffers from is assuming that all that we don't know is rubbish. We urge you to keep an open mind. If all we've managed to do through this book is to make you question everything, then we've succeeded in what we set out to do.

Now back to pasting that smile on and start moving. And spread it all around.

Keep miling and smiling!

Acknowledgements

3rd August 21

Dear Rajat,

Wow! I got your letter (mentioning about the book) today and reading it was remembering similar episodes in my training. It was clear that I had to create our own hospital, so that we could practice medicine – the way we wanted to – not their way. That clarity has never diminished in me for a moment. So I'm still (after 51 years) trying to build our radical free hospital in our poorest state: West Virginia. We will have all the healing arts.

    Follow your dreams.
    Whee!!

Yours,
Patch
(Dr Patch Adams)

Family: Aria Player, Jayden Player, Meena Player, V.S. Chauhan, Viren Chauhan, Harsheath Chauhan and Nidhi Chauhan.

Production Family: Milee Ashwarya, Nicholas Rixon, Radhika Agarwal, Shivangi Kanodia, Archana Rajgopal, Saksham Garg, Rinjini Mitra and Priya Iyer-Vyas.

The Three Musketeers: Voltaire, Vincent van Gogh and Richard Feynman.

Friends, Mentors (Known or Unknown) and Colleagues: Champa Dhakpa, Dr Hardev Singh Girn, Surgeon Captain Dr Jagbir Singh Nagra (retired), Dr R.P. Pai, Dr Kshitij Malik, Jaidhar Vashist, Dr Patch Adams, Dr Peter L. Gregory, Dr Roderic Macdonald, Dr Jens Foell, Prof. Timothy Noakes, Prof. Karim Khan, Dr Richard Stretch, Prof. Panteleimon (Paddy) Ekkekakis, Dr Kelly McGonigal, Dr Mark Steven Woolley, Purnima Sahai, Shashwati, Preeti Singh, Dr Divya Parashar, Dr Ivan Tyrrell, Prateek Gupta, Kieron Berry, Commander Abhilash Tomy, Dr Deepak Srivastav, Subhash Rana and Prof. Matthew Walker.

Others Mentioned in the Book: Dr Nidhi Dhawan, Shikha Pahwa, Dr Raju Easwaran, Amit Kshirsagar, Dr Amit Srivastava, Dr Arvind Bhateja, Dr Anjali Kumar, Madhav Kumar, Dr Anant Joshi, Dr Gurinder Bedi, Dr Erika Patel, Ray Sánchez, Sharon Gayter, Dr Siri Terjesen, Dr Priyanka Mantri, Dr Linda George, Aparna Ramachandra, Dr William 'Bill' Andrews, Herrick 'Rick' Andrews, Dr Bradley Elliot and Christine Pemberton.

MoveMint Medicine Podcast: Kevin Wyld, Dr Aashish Contractor, Dr C.N. Radhakrishnan, Dr Surabhi Kalita, Dr Meenakshi Hariharan, Dr Gurmeet Soni Bhalla, Dr Hemant Shirdi Rana, Dr Aditya Daftary, Mandeep Singh, Dr Tvisha Parikh, Dr Shashidhar Tatavarthy, Dr Deepak Chaudhary, Dr Anindita Bhateja, Dr Abhay Nene, Dr Kinjal Bhat, Dr Amish Vora, Dr Sangeeta Saikia, Dr Neelu Khanna, Dr Pankaj Surange, Dr Shekar Ramineni, Dr Hemanth Vudayaraju, Dr Kamna Ahuja, Dr Rushad Shroff, Dr Madhumathi Sanjay, Dr Raja Rami Reddy, Dr G. Swarnalatha, Dr Vinay Tiwary, Dr Ramakrishnan A.S., Dr Sonali Chaturvedi, Dr Sanjay Suryakant Kate, Dr Lakshmi Sundar, Dr Raj Kumar, Dr Sanjay Dhawan, Dr Pranav Desai, Kieran Lowe, Dr (Col) Rajesh Adhau, Dr Harpreet Kour, Dr Akshith, Dr Anil Chauhan and David Poulter.

High Talk Panel: Daniel Phuntsog, Ayesha Billimoria, Sonia Jain, Swaty Singh Malik, Shiva Keshavan, Charles Assisi, Ashish Kasodekar, Raj Vadgama, Jyotsana Rawat, Chetan Sehgal, Reeti Sahai, Gautam Sood, Ripu Daman, Santhosh Padmanabhan, Alfredo Miranda, Sandeep Mall, Gagandeep Kaur, Jagmohan, Shibani Gharat, Sujata Kelkar, Tanvi Lad, Mukul Oberoi and Alatakshi Gosain.

Changed Names: Mahender Shah, Vidur Thakar, Nisha, Rajeev Lingaraju, Priyanka Narang, Rupinder Chopra, and Ajay and Pooja Mehra.

Notes

Introduction

1   Adams, Patch, *Gesundheit!: Bringing Good Health to You, the Medical System, and Society through Physician Service, Complementary Therapies, Humor, and Joy*, Healing Arts Press, 1998.

2   Michôd, D. (director), 2017, *War Machine,* Plan B Entertainment, Blue-Tongue Films.

3   See Leonardo da Vinci, Quotes, Quotable Quotes n.d., Good Reads, accessed 16 January 2022, https://www.goodreads.com/quotes/112565-principles-for-the-development-of-a-complete-mind-study-the.

4   Adams, P., 'Gesundheit: Patch Adams at TEDx Utrecht University', TED, May 2012, https://youtu.be/Maw4Xg-6RAw.

5   Dictionary, O.E., 1 December 2021, OED Online, retrieved from Oxford University Press, https://www.oed.com/view/Entry/123027?rskey=AulWDq&result=2#eid.

6   Ibid.

7   Ibid.

Chapter 1: Dream, Life and Patch

1   Sallis R. et al., 'Physical inactivity is associated with a higher risk for severe COVID-19 outcomes: a study in 48,440 adult patients', *British Journal of Sports Medicine*, 2021; 0:1–8, doi:10.1136/bjsports-2021-104080.

2   Girard, F. (director), 2015, *Boychoir*, Informant Films.

3   Kolata, Gina, '5 Decades of Warnings Fail to Get Americans Moving', *New York Times*, 10 September 2002.

4   See https://twitter.com/ekkekakis/status/1441503875375173633?s=21 (tweeted on 25 September 2021).

5   See https://twitter.com/mescottdouglas/status/1441505340000923648?s=21.

6   See https://twitter.com/ekkekakis/status/1441503875375173633?s=21 (tweeted on 25 September 2021).

7   Solomon, A., 2016, 'Literature about medicine may be all that can save us', *Guardian*, 22 April 2016, Accessed 16 January 2022, https://www.theguardian.com/books/2016/apr/22/literature-about-medicine-may-be-all-that-can-save-us.

8   Shadyac, T. (director), 1998, *Patch Adams*, Blue Wolf, Bungalow 78 Productions, Farrell/Minoff.

9   Ibid.

10 Adams, P., 'Gesundheit: Patch Adams at TEDx Utrecht University', TED, May 2012, https://youtu.be/Maw4Xg-6RAw.

11 McGonigal, Kelly, *The Joy of Movement: How Exercise Helps Us Find Happiness, Hope, Connection, and Courage*, Avery (an imprint of Penguin Random House), 2019.

12 Ekkekakis, P., 'Exercise Psychology: Promoting Exercise By Promising That You Will Only Have to Do "A Little Bit"', YouTube, January 2020.

13 Bauman, A.E., Kamala, M. and Reid, R.S. et al., 'An evidence-based assessment of the impact of the Olympic Games on population levels of physical activity', *Lancet*, 2021, 398: 456–464, https://doi.org/10.1016/S0140-6736(21)01165-X.

14 Adams, Patch., *Gesundheit!: Bringing Good Health to You, the Medical System, and Society through Physician Service, Complementary Therapies, Humor, and Joy*, Healing Arts Press, 1998.

15 Adams, P., 'Gesundheit: Patch Adams at TEDx Utrecht University', TED, May 2012, https://youtu.be/Maw4Xg-6RAw.

16 Ibid.

17 Adams, Patch., *Gesundheit!: Bringing Good Health to You, the Medical System, and Society through Physician Service, Complementary Therapies, Humor, and Joy*, Healing Arts Press, 1998.

18 Ibid.

19 Adams, P., 'Gesundheit: Patch Adams at TEDx Utrecht University', TED, May 2012, https://youtu.be/Maw4Xg-6RAw.

20 Adams, Patch., *Gesundheit!: Bringing Good Health to You, the Medical System, and Society through Physician Service, Complementary Therapies, Humor, and Joy*, Healing Arts Press, 1998.

21 Ibid.

22 Ibid.

23 Málaga, G., Gayoso D. and Vásquez N., 'Empathy in medical students of a private university in Lima, Peru: A descriptive study', *Medwave*, 25 May 2020, 20(4):e7905, Spanish, English, doi: 10.5867/medwave.2020.04.7905, PMID: 32469857.

24 Tariq, N., Rasheed T. and Tavakol M., 'A Quantitative Study of Empathy in Pakistani Medical Students: A Multicentered Approach', *Journal of Primary Care & Community Health*, October 2017, 8(4):294–99, doi: 10.1177/2150131917716233, Epub: 23 June 2017, PMID: 28645236; PMCID: PMC5932734; and Shaheen, A., Mahmood M.A., Zia-Ul-Miraj M. and Ahmad M., 'Empathy levels among undergraduate medical students in Pakistan, a cross sectional study using Jefferson scale of physician empathy', *Journal of Pakistan Medical Association*, July 2020; 70(7):1149–53; doi: 10.5455/JPMA.301593, PMID: 32799264.

25 Williams, B., Sadasivan S. and Kadirvelu A., 'Malaysian Medical Students' Self-reported Empathy: A Cross-sectional Comparative

Study', *Medical Journal of Malaysia*, April 2015, 70(2):76–80, PMID: 26162381.

26 Akgün, Ö., Akdeniz M., Kavukcu E. and Avcı H.H., 'Medical Students' Empathy Level Differences by Medical Year, Gender, and Specialty Interest in Akdeniz University', *Journal of Medical Education and Curricular Development*, 31 July 2020, 7:2382120520940658, doi: 10.1177/2382120520940658, PMID: 32923670, PMCID: PMC7446269.

27 Wen, D., Ma X., Li H., Liu Z., Xian B. and Liu Y., 'Empathy in Chinese medical students: psychometric characteristics and differences by gender and year of medical education', *BMC Medical Education*, 23 September 2013,13:130, doi: 10.1186/1472-6920-13-130, PMID: 24053330, PMCID: PMC3848862; and Ye, X., Guo H., Xu Z. and Xiao H., 'Empathy variation of undergraduate medical students after early clinical contact: a cross-sectional study in China', *BMJ Open,* 19 July 2020, 10(7):e035690, doi: 10.1136/bmjopen-2019-035690, PMID: 32690511, PMCID: PMC7371130.

28 Chen, D.C., Kirshenbaum, D.S., Yan J., Kirshenbaum E. and Aseltine R.H., 'Characterizing changes in student empathy throughout medical school', *Medical Teacher*, 2012, 34(4):305-11, doi: 10.3109/0142159X.2012.644600, PMID: 22455699; and Chen, D., Lew R., Hershman W. and Orlander J., 'A cross-sectional measurement of medical student empathy', *Journal of General Internal Medicine,* October 2007, 22(10):1434-8, doi: 10.1007/s11606-007-0298-x, Epub: 26 July 2007, PMID: 17653807, PMCID: PMC2305857; and Hojat, M., Vergare M.J., Maxwell K., Brainard G., Herrine S.K., Isenberg G.A., Veloski J. and Gonnella J.S., 'The devil is in the third year: a longitudinal study of erosion of empathy in medical school', *Academic Medicine,* September 2009, 84(9):1182-91, doi: 10.1097/ACM.0b013e3181b17e55, Erratum in: *Academic Medicine,* November 2009, 84(11):1616, PMID: 19707055.

29 Rezayat, A.A., Shahini N., Asl H.T., Jarahi L., Behdani F., Shojaei S.R.H. and Abadi J.S.A., 'Empathy score among

medical students in Mashhad, Iran: study of the Jefferson Scale of Physician Empathy', *Electron Physician Journal*, 25 July 2018, 10(7):7101-06, doi: 10.19082/7101, PMID: 30128102, PMCID: PMC6092132; and Shariat, S.V. and Habibi M., 'Empathy in Iranian medical students: measurement model of the Jefferson scale of empathy', *Medical Teacher*, 2013, 35(1):e913-8, doi: 10.3109/0142159X.2012.714881, Epub: 3 September 2012, PMID: 22938682; and Hizomi Arani, R., Naji Z., Moradi A., Shariat S.V., Mirzamohamadi S. and Salamati P., 'Comparison of empathy with patients between first-year and last-year medical students of Tehran University of Medical Sciences', *BMC Medical Education*, 30 August 2021, 21(1):460, doi: 10.1186/s12909-021-02897-0, PMID: 34461865, PMCID: PMC8406781.

30 Santiago, L.M., Rosendo I., Coutinho M.L., Maurício K.S., Neto I. and Simões J.A., 'Comparing empathy in medical students of two Portuguese medicine schools', *BMC Medical Education*, 13 May 2020, 20(1):153, doi: 10.1186/s12909-020-02034-3, PMID: 32404095, PMCID: PMC7218824.

31 Dashash, M. and Boubou M., 'Measurement of empathy among health professionals during Syrian crisis using the Syrian empathy scale', *BMC Medical Education*, 29 July 2021, 21(1):409, doi: 10.1186/s12909-021-02835-0, PMID: 34325698, PMCID: PMC8319893.

32 Biswas, B., Haldar A., Dasgupta A., Mallick N. and Karmakar A., 'An Epidemiological Study on Empathy and Its Correlates: A Cross-sectional Assessment among Medical Students of a Government Medical College of India', *Indian Journal of Psychological Medicine*, July–August 2018, 40(4):364-369, doi: 10.4103/IJPSYM.IJPSYM_109_18, PMID: 30093748, PMCID: PMC6065120; and Shashikumar, R., Chaudhary R., Ryali V.S., Bhat P.S., Srivastava K., Prakash J. and Basannar D., 'Cross sectional assessment of empathy among undergraduates from a medical college', *Medical Journal Armed Forces India*, April 2014, 70(2):179-85, doi: 10.1016/j.mjafi.2014.02.005, Epub:

12 April 2014, PMID: 24843209, PMCID: PMC4017208; and Shashikumar, R., Agarwal K., Mohammad A. and Kaushik C., 'Multiple cross-sectional assessments of empathy in medical undergraduate students'. *Industrial Psychiatry Journal*, January–June 2021, 30(1):147-52, doi: 10.4103/ipj.ipj_63_21, Epub: June 2021, PMID: 34483540, PMCID: PMC8395536.

33 N.V.R. Krishnamacharya, The Mahabharata, Tirupati: Tirumala Tirupati Devasthanams, 1983.

34 Indian society is divided into groups based on their lifestyle, social status and occupation. Brahmins happens to be on top of that pyramid in status.

35 Wachowskis, T. (director), 2003, *The Matrix Reloaded*, Village Roadshow Pictures, NPV Entertainment, Silver Pictures.

36 See Maya Angelou, Quotes, Quotable Quotes n.d., Good Reads, accessed 16 January 2022, https://www.goodreads.com/quotes/5934-i-ve-learned-that-people-will-forget-what-you-said-people.

Chapter 2: The Three Musketeers (Don't 'Dis' Them)

1 Leighton, R., *What Do You Care What Other People Think?: Further Adventures of a Curious Character*, W.W. Norton, 1988.

2 Tsiaras, A., 'Conception to birth – visualized', TED, November 2011, https://youtu.be/fKyljukBE70.

3 'Picosecond', 2021, retrieved on 12 January 2022, https://en.m.wikipedia.org/wiki/Picosecond.

4 Dictionary, O.E., 1 December 2021, OED Online, retrieved from Oxford University Press, https://www.oed.com/view/Entry/123027?rskey=AulWDq&result=2#eid.

5 'Chronology of the universe', 2022, retrieved on 12 January 2022.

6 Fuqua, A. (director), 2007, *Shooter*, di Bonaventura Pictures.

7 Audi Technology Portal, 2021, chassis, 9 September 2021, https://www.audi-technology-portal.de/en/chassis.

Chapter 3: Psychology

1   See Charlie Chaplin, Quotes, Quotable Quotes n.d., Good
     Reads, accessed 16 January 2022, https://www.goodreads.com/
     quotes/616577-we-think-too-much-and-feel-too-little-more-
     than.

2   Charlie Chaplin, Quotes, Quotable Quotes n.d., Good Reads,
     accessed   16   January   2022,   https://www.goodreads.com/
     quotes/1333387-simplicity-is-not-a-simple-thing.

3   Natsuki Takaya, Quotes, Quotable Quotes n.d., Good Reads,
     accessed   16   January   2022,   https://www.goodreads.com/
     quotes/222519-it-s-all-very-simple-but-maybe-because-it-s-so-
     simple.

4   Information shared via Zoom on 28 October 2021.

5   Patient name used with her consent; written communication to Dr
     Rajat Chauhan dated 31 December 2020.

6   Dr Divya Parashar is a clinical and rehabilitation psychologist with
     over twenty years of experience. She is the former head, psychology
     department, Indian Spinal Injuries Centre, New Delhi. She works
     with individuals to enhance their potential and function at their
     best, whatever be their illness or disability.

7   Preeti Singh in written communication to Dr Rajat Chauhan
     dated 12 September 2020.

8   Preeti Singh in written communication to Dr Rajat Chauhan
     dated 25 December 2020.

Chapter 4: Psychological Needs (The Human Givens)

1   Human Givens is the name of a theory in psychotherapy formulated
     in the UK, first outlined by Joe Griffin and Ivan Tyrrell in the
     late 1990s and amplified in the 2003 book, *Human Givens: A New
     Approach to Emotional Health and Clear Thinking,* Human Givens,
     2021, retrieved on 12 January 2022, https://en.m.wikipedia.org/
     wiki/Human_givens.

2   Online video discussion with authors on 11 October 2020.

3   Mann, M. (director), 1995, *Heat*, Regency Enterprises, Forward Pass.

4   The Run & Bee running mentoring programme was put together by Dr Rajat Chauhan and his team in September 2020.

5   Scott, T. (director), 1986, *Top Gun*, Don Simpson/Jerry Bruckheimer Films.

6   Waitzkin, J., *The Art of Learning: An Inner Journey to Optimal Performance*, Free Press, May 2007.

7   Zemeckis, R. (director), 1994, *Forrest Gump*, The Tisch Company.

8   Chandan, A. (director), 2022, *Laal Singh Chaddha*, Aamir Khan Productions, Viacom18 Studios.

Chapter 5: Psy-Phy: The Psychology of Movement

1   Adams, P., 'Gesundheit: Patch Adams at TEDx Utrecht University', TED, May 2012, https://youtu.be/Maw4Xg-6RAw.

2   Ekkekakis, P., 'Exercise hedonics: Pleasure and displeasure responses to exercise', American College of Sports Medicine Brown Bag Series in Science Webinar, March 2018, https://youtu.be/3oZKxHmPgAM.

3   Department for Education, 'Behaviour and discipline in schools', advice for headteachers and school staff, February 2014, www.gov.uk/government/publications.

4   Ragra-patti means rolling on the ground.

5   Surveys conducted on https://twitter.com/drrajatchauhan/status/1304310710797651968?s=20 on 11 September 2020 and on https://twitter.com/drrajatchauhan/status/1400701927898312704?s=20 on 4 June 2021.

6   'Perceived Importance of Physical Activity and Walkable Neighborhoods Among US Adults', 2017, published in December 2020.

7   'Brits "dying not to do exercise"', 17 September 2007, BBC News, http://news.bbc.co.uk/1/hi/health/6994632.stm.

8 Ekkekakis, P., 'Exercise Psychology: Promoting exercise by promising that you will only have to do "a little bit"', YouTube, January 2020.

9 Ibid.

10 Ibid.

11 McGonigal, Kelly, *The Joy of Movement: How Exercise Helps Us Find Happiness, Hope, Connection, and Courage*, Avery (an imprint of Penguin Random House), 2019.

12 'Daring rescue ends Navy Commander Abhilash Tomy's 70-hour ordeal, wife still waits for phone call', *Hindustan Times*, 25 September 2018, https://www.hindustantimes.com/india-news/daring-rescue-ends-navy-commander-abhilash-tomy-s-70-hour-ordeal-wife-still-waits-for-phone-call/story-PSB4SVvhL3ilStQbuyndIO_amp.html.

13 Ekkekakis, P., 'Exercise Psychology: Promoting exercise by promising that you will only have to do "a little bit"', YouTube, January 2020.

14 Ibid.

Chapter 6: Sleepin' It Off

1 Srivastava, D., 'World Sleep Day 2021 - India Celebrates Sleep #Webinar 1 - Why You Can't Sleep', https://youtu.be/6m_S9pao9No.

2 Ibid.

3 Bon Jovi, J., 1993, 'I'll Sleep When I'm Dead', Keep the Faith, Bob Rock, https://youtu.be/ts-e0uZfooQ.

4 Oliver S.J., Costa R.J., Laing S.J., Bilzon J.L. and Walsh N.P., 'One night of sleep deprivation decreases treadmill endurance performance', *European Journal of Applied Physiology*, September 2009, 107(2):155-61, doi: 10.1007/s00421-009-1103-9, Epub: 20 June 2009, PMID: 19543909.

5 Philips Global Sleep Survey 2021, 17 March 2021, Philips, 23 August 2021, https://www.philips.co.in/a-w/about/news/archive/standard/about/news/press/2021/20211703-philips-india-sleep-

survey-2021-reveals-that-indian-adults-slept-more-during-covid-19-pandemic.html; and Verma, Y., 'World Sleep Day 2021 - India Celebrates Sleep #Webinar 1 - Why You Can't Sleep', https://youtu.be/6m_S9pao9No.

6   Ibid.

7   Tamar Sofer, Matthew O. Goodman, Suzanne M. Bertisch and Susan Redline, 'Longer sleep improves cardiovascular outcomes: time to make sleep a priority', *European Heart Journal*, Volume 42, Issue 34, 7 September 2021, pp. 3358–60, https://doi.org/10.1093/eurheartj/ehab248.

8   Ekirch, R., *At Day's Close: Night in Times Past*, W.W. Norton & Company, illustrated edition, 17 October 2006.

9   Ekirch, A.R., 'Segmented sleep in preindustrial societies', SLEEP, 2016, 39(3):715–16.

10 Walker, M., *Why We Sleep: Unlocking the Power of Sleep and Dreams*, Scribner, illustrated edition, 19 June 2018.

11 Ibid.

12 Alison Wimms, Holger Woehrle, Sahisha Ketheeswaran, Dinesh Ramanan and Jeffery Armitstead, 'Obstructive Sleep Apnea in Women: Specific Issues and Interventions', *BioMed Research International*, Vol. 2016, article ID: 1764837, nine pages, 2016, https://doi.org/10.1155/2016/1764837.

13 Srivastava, D., 'World Sleep Day 2021 - India Celebrates Sleep #Webinar 1 - Why You Can't Sleep', https://youtu.be/6m_S9pao9No.

14 Walker, M., *Why We Sleep: Unlocking the Power of Sleep and Dreams*, Scribner, illustrated edition, 19 June 2018.

15 Ibid.

16 Ibid.

Chapter 7: *MoveMint* Nutrition

1   Sanderson, Helen, Renfrew, Jane M., Prance, Ghillean and Nesbitt, Mark (eds), *The Cultural History of Plants*, Routledge, 2005, p. 106.

2   Witkamp, R.V., 2018, 'Let thy food be thy medicine....when possible', *European Journal of Pharmacology, 836*, 102-14.

3   Maffetone, P. and Khopkar M., 'The overfat pandemic in India', *Global Epidemic Obesity*, 2018, 6:2, http://dx.doi. org/10.7243/2052-5966-6-2.

4   Luhar, S., Timæus I.M., Jones R., Cunningham S. and Patel S.A. et al., 2020, 'Forecasting the prevalence of overweight and obesity in India to 2040', *PLOS One*, 15(2): e0229438, https://doi. org/10.1371/journal.pone.0229438.

5   Sarlio-Lähteenkorva, S. and Winkler J.T., 'Could a sugar tax help combat obesity?' *BMJ*, 2015, 351 :h4047, doi:10.1136/bmj.h4047.

6   *Sun* UK, 6 November 2021, 'HO HO NO Coffee chain Christmas drinks contain up to whopping 63 GRAMS of sugar', retrieved from The Sun Online: https://www.thesun.co.uk/health/16657485/ coffee-chain-christmas-drinks-sugar/.

7   Patient name used with her consent, obtained on 4 January 2022; information shared with Dr Rajat Chauhan on 15 February 2021.

8   Price, Weston A., *Nutrition and Physical Degeneration: A Comparison of Primitive and Modern Diets and Their Effects, 1939*, Paul B. Hoeber, Inc; Medical Book Department of Harper & Brothers.

Chapter 8: MSK: 'M'ake 'S'ure You 'K'now

1   According to the Mahabharata, Duryodhan's mother Gandhari wanted to use the mystic power of her eyes to make his body indestructible. She asked him to bathe and appear naked before her so she could do so. While on his way to see his mother, Duryodhan bumped into Lord Krishna, who mocked his state of undress. An embarrassed Duryodhan covered his private parts, thus leaving a part of his body weak.

2   Chauhan, R.P., 26 March 2020, 'MoveMint Medicine', retrieved from YouTube: https://youtube.com/c/MoveMintMedicine.

3   See YouTube channel: MoveMint Medicine, https://youtube. com/c/MoveMintMedicine.

Chapter 9: Women's Health

1   Saxena, G.S., 2018, 'Position of Women In Vedic, Post-Vedic, British, And Contemporary India', *International Journal of Legal Developments And Allied Issues*, 372–80.

2   Morris, D., *The Naked Woman: A Study of the Female Body*, 2011, Vintage Digital, New Edition.

3   Power, M., 2008, 'Sex differences in fat storage, fat metabolism, and the health risks from obesity: Possible evolutionary origins', *British Journal of Nutrition*, *99*(5), 931–40.

4   Badwater Ultramarathon describes itself as 'the world's toughest foot race'. It is a 135-mile course starting at 282 feet below sea level in the Badwater Basin, in California's Death Valley, and ending at an elevation of 8360 feet at Whitney Portal, the trailhead to Mount Whitney; Badwater Ultramarathon, 2021, retrieved on 12 January 2022, https://en.m.wikipedia.org/wiki/Badwater_Ultramarathon.

5   Khardung La, 2002, https://en.m.wikipedia.org/wiki/Khardung_La; and Umling La, 2021, retrieved on 12 January 2022, https://en.m.wikipedia.org/wiki/Umling_La.

6   Williams, F., 'Desperate Housewife Stalks Male Supermodel in Sports Death March', Outside online, 1 October 2005, https://www.outsideonline.com/health/running/desperate-housewife-stalks-male-supermodel-sports-death-march/.

7   Constantina Diță, 2020, retrieved on 12 January 2022, https://en.m.wikipedia.org/wiki/Special:History/Constantina_Diță.

8   'Siri Terjesen ('93)—Cross Country and Track', Revere Schools, 2015,   https://www.revereschools.org/cms/lib02/OH01001097/Centricity/Domain/202/2015%20Revere%20Athletic%20HOF%20Profiles--Siri%20Terjesen.pdf.

9   Damian Best, Alison Avenell and Siladitya Bhattacharya, November 2017, 'How effective are weight-loss interventions for improving fertility in women and men who are overweight or obese? A systematic review and meta-analysis of the evidence' *Human Reproduction Update, 23*(6), 681–705.

10 MoveMint Medicine podcast, 7 April 2020, https://youtu.be/7F5TxEr3_qk.

11 Ibid.

12 'This Girl Can', 1 January 2022, Homepage, retrieved from This Girl Can: https://www.thisgirlcan.co.uk/.

13 Personal communication with Dr Rajat Chauhan via email on 26 November 2020.

14 Personal testimony to Dr Rajat Chauhan.

15 25 Maya Angelou Quotes To Inspire Your Life, Goalcast, accessed 16 January 2022, https://www.goalcast.com/maya-angelou-quotes-to-inspire-your-life/.

Chapter 10: Ageing Well

1 Interviewed by Dr Rajat Chauhan on Zoom on 20 December 2020.

2 Ibid.

3 Ibid.

4 World Health Organization, 'Global recommendations on physical activity for health', 1 January 2010, https://www.who.int/dietphysicalactivity/factsheet_recommendations.

5 Kim, K., Choi, S. and Hwang S.E. et al., 'Changes in exercise frequency and cardiovascular outcomes in older adults', *European Heart Journal*, Volume 41, Issue 15, 14 April 2020, pp. 1490–99, https://doi.org/10.1093/eurheartj/ehz768.

6 Roberts, W.O., 'Running causes knee osteoarthritis: myth or misunderstanding', *British Journal of Sports Medicine*, 2018, 52:142.

7 Personal communication with Dr Rajat Chauhan.

8 'Exercise and aging: Can you walk away from Father Time', *Harvard Health*, Harvard Health Publishing, Harvard Medical School, 9 March 2014.

Conclusion

1 Bieber, J., Levin B. and Sheeran E., 2015, 'Love Yourself, Purpose, Benny Blanco. https://youtu.be/oyEuk8j8imI.